Promoting a Comprehensive School Health Program

Judy R. Jonas
Texas Comprehensive School Health Initiative

Gay James
Southwest Texas State University

Edward Manigold
Texas Association of School Administrators

Glencoe
McGraw-Hill

New York, New York   Columbus, Ohio   Woodland Hills, California   Peoria, Illinois

About the Authors

Judy R. Jonas, R.D., M.Ed., is the project director for the Texas Comprehensive School Health Initiative (TCSHI). With a background in nutrition, health promotion, and community organization, Ms. Jonas has worked with numerous professional organizations to facilitate the development of partnerships for healthy schools. In addition to coalition-building activities, she assists in organizing the state's annual school health promotion conference, Texas *ALL WELL,* currently in its seventh year.

Gay James, Ph.D., is assistant professor of health at Southwest Texas State University and an associate director of the AIDS Consortium of Texas, Colleges and Universities. Dr. James is active on many councils working on comprehensive school health issues and has served on the *ALL WELL* planning team since its inception seven years ago.

Edward Manigold, Ed.D., is the associate executive director for programs and professional development for the Texas Association of School Administrators. An active leader in public education for the past thirty years, Dr. Manigold has served as an administrator for a local school district, a regional education service center, and the state education agency. He conducts extensive training in school leadership and governance issues.

Glencoe/McGraw-Hill

A Division of The McGraw-Hill Companies

Printed in the United States of America.

Send all inquiries to:
Glencoe/McGraw-Hill
21600 Oxnard Street, Suite 500
Woodland Hills, CA 91367

ISBN 0-02-652745-6 Promoting a Comprehensive School Health Program

7 8 9 10 11 12 045 04 03 02 01 00 99

Promoting a Comprehensive School Health Program

Table of Contents

Part 1: Recognizing the Need for a Comprehensive School Health Program
Introduction 1
Purpose of This Booklet 2
Why Is a Comprehensive Approach to School Health Needed? 3
A Collaborative Approach to School Health 4
Barriers 5
The Goal: Collaboration 5
Building Teamwork 6
The Cost of Prevention 6
What Are the Health Facts in Your Community? 9
Building an Approach 11
Comprehensive School Health — Informal Survey 12
Summary and Next Steps 15
Getting Started 15

Part 2: Planning a Comprehensive School Health Program
Introduction 16
Site-Based Decision Making and a Vision 16
Developing a Shared Vision 17
Desired Results for Students 18
Identifying Desired Results 19
Assessing Current Conditions 19
Completing the Comprehensive School Health Survey 19
Selecting Areas for Action 19
Summary and Next Steps 20

Part 3: Implementing a Comprehensive School Health Program
Introduction 21
Taking Action 21
Brainstorming Major Problems 22
Understanding Causes and Effects 24
Action for Program Improvement 25
Working Your Plan 26
Measuring Progress 26
Summary 27

Appendixes
Appendix A: Comprehensive School Health Survey 28
Appendix B: Sample Action Plan 41
Appendix C: Standards for Comprehensive School Health Programs 42
Appendix D: School Health Advisory Council Evaluation Checklist 49
Appendix E: Resource Directory 50

Bibliography 63
Credits 64

Part 1

Recognizing the Need for a Comprehensive School Health Program

Introduction

No institution touches the lives of more citizens than the education system. This system, however, is faced with an alarming number of problems related to the physical and mental well-being of the children served. These problems may stem from the child's inadequate education, poor nutrition, peer pressure, and economic and social conditions or inadequate parenting. Everyone pays when health problems are neglected, and everyone benefits when efforts are focused on prevention. Each community, each school, and each family must share responsibility for developing a school health partnership.

This booklet is divided into three parts. Part 1 highlights the need for a collaborative and comprehensive approach and offers a description of the elements necessary for an effective program. Part 2 offers tools and techniques to assist in developing a shared vision, assessing local needs, and selecting priority areas for action. Part 3 contains information to help move the ideas into action.

Problems

- An unhealthy child is unable to learn and is at greater risk for failure in school. School failure has lifelong negative consequences for the child as well as for society. Children who fail in school will not be as employable as those who succeed. In 1992 the unemployment rate for those who dropped out (11.4 percent) was nearly twice that of those who graduated from high school but did not go on to college (6.8 percent). The median income of those completing high school was nearly double that of high school dropouts (1).*
- A majority of prison inmates are high school dropouts. In one state it costs approximately $13,000 per year to support an 18-year-old in a state prison, while it costs approximately $12,000 per year to attend a state-supported university (2, 3).
- Every five years our nation's bill for health care doubles. By 1995 it will reach nearly $1 trillion. However, one in every five of America's children lived below the poverty line in 1991, with nearly 13 percent having no health insurance and more than 15 percent having no regular health care (4).

** See data source in Bibliography on page 63.*

As the saying goes, "pay me now or pay me later." Prevention is significantly more cost-effective than treatment. Each family, each school, each community, all citizens must share responsibility for developing solutions that result in a school health partnership. Following are steps to take.

Solutions

- Empower parents, communities, schools, and students.
- Mobilize resources within one complete and efficient network.
- Influence a wide variety of stakeholders.
- Make health education and services a part of the school climate.
- Focus attention on healthy schools as a priority.
- View wellness as part of the school environment.

The future of our children rests upon the realization that "at risk" doesn't have to mean "doomed." Risk and degrees of risk can be changed. Health problems affect educational progress. Prevention lowers long-term costs.

Payoffs That Are a Result of Comprehensive School Health Planning

- Positive self-images
- Skills in interpersonal relationships
- Coping skills
- Self-responsibility
- Potential for becoming secure, knowledgeable adults
- Increased capacity for becoming productive taxpayers

In the face of the immediate challenges to schools and healthy youth, parents, schools and communities must mobilize resources and coordinate efforts. Together, we can succeed in building healthy students and healthy schools.

Purpose of This Booklet

Because of the critical nature of the health needs of students, and because learning is so closely tied to health, children's physical and mental well-being warrant priority attention. This booklet is a tool that can help call attention to the underlying causes of poor health and welfare of children and adolescents. It is intended to assist schools in strengthening existing programs to more fully meet the expectations of school staff, parents, and community members in shaping successful, healthy students.

A comprehensive school health (CSH) program is an organized set of policies, procedures, and activities designed to protect and promote the health and well-being of students and staff. A school health program has traditionally included school health instruction, health services, and a healthy school environment. An expanded definition also includes physical education, counseling and guidance, school food service, employee health promotion, and school/community partnerships for healthy students (5).

Perhaps the term *collaborative school health program* would be more descriptive, because the factors that influence the healthy development of young people lie both within and outside the school's sphere of influence. We cannot expect to build healthy lifestyles for future generations by offering students occasional lectures or assemblies on disease prevention, by placing more emphasis on competitive sports than on lifetime fitness, or by teaching healthy nutrition guidelines in the classroom while providing unhealthy choices in vending machines and school cafeterias. Instead, a well organized program of services and education is needed both within the school and outside of the school.

The schools in your community already have the basic ingredients for an effective comprehensive school health program. This booklet is intended to help your community's schools tap into a system of health programming already in place. Most schools have health instruction and physical education classes, counseling and nursing services, substance abuse prevention programs, special education programs, and programs linked with Departments of Health,

Human Services, and volunteer health agencies. Schools also may have a site-based decision-making committee or campus improvement committee comprising teachers, school staff, parents, community members, and business representatives. In addition to site-based decision making and campus improvement committees, many schools have dropout prevention committees and school/community drug prevention committees. Such committes are not mutually exclusive. Plans to promote academic success must include efforts to promote healthy students as well.

The *primary* purpose of this booklet is to help schools gain support for strengthening programs and services that are designed to address locally determined health and education priorities. This booklet is also a response to the U.S. Health and Human Services document *Healthy People 2000,* which outlines the health promotion and disease objectives that are vital for a healthy future (6). Schools have a significant role in helping meet over 100 of the objectives. Working together, school personnel, parents, state and county agencies, volunteer organizations, and other community members can provide young people with the knowledge and skills needed to help them become tomorrow's healthy, productive adults.

School systems are not responsible for meeting every need of their students, but where the need directly affects learning, the school must meet the challenge. So it is with health.

(Carnegie Council on Adolescent Development)

Why Is a Comprehensive Approach to School Health Needed?

Two major shifts have changed the public school's responsibility for students' health. First, dramatic changes have occurred in the structure of the American family and the demographics of the school-age population. As a result, the school environment has changed significantly. Consider the following changes in behavior problems that affect the educational environment.

Student Behavior/School Environment Problems Through Time

40 Years Ago

Talking
Chewing gum
Making noise
Running in the halls
Being out of place in line
Wearing improper clothing
Not using wastebasket
Having a messy locker
Holding hands
Being tardy

Today

Gang violence
Alcohol and other drug abuse
Weapons
Drug dealing
Pregnancy and unwed mothers
Gang colors and clothing
Suicide
Sexual harassment
Assault of teachers and students
Dropouts

These are sample behavior problems, and are not reflective of an actual survey.

Second, the leading causes of disease and death in the United States have shifted from infectious diseases to behavior-related chronic diseases. According to the Centers for Disease Control and Prevention and the Bureau of Health Statistics, about half (48 percent) of the deaths in the United States are caused by factors that are directly related to lifestyle choices.

Causes of Death

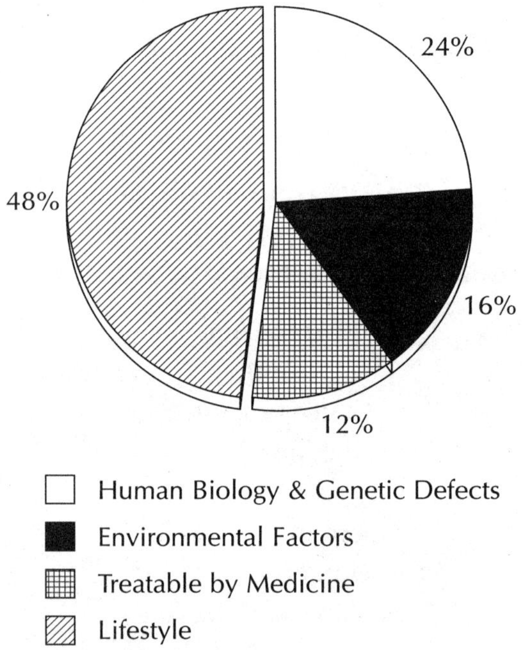

Source: Centers for Disease Control and Prevention

Children pattern their actions after peers and adults. Poor choices in social environment and/or specific lifestyles that lead to preventable health problems often occur during youth. It is more difficult to change or influence an adult's learned behavior than it is to foster healthy habits in the young. That is why a collaborative and comprehensive school health program is so essential.

A Collaborative Approach to School Health

Schools cannot do it alone. School-age children spend about 1,225 hours in school each year (7 hours per day x 175 days). Approximately 21 percent of their time each week is spent in school. This means that during the school year, or August to June, about 79 percent of school-age children's time is spent at home or in places *other than* school. While the school can have a great deal of influence on students during the time they are there, many other factors influence and shape student behavior and lifestyle. What are the factors contributing to a student's physical and mental health and academic success?

Factors Inside the School

- Curriculum
- Teachers and staff members
- Instructional arrangements and methodology
- Instructional materials
- Amount of time spent on task
- Schedule for classes/subjects
- School support services, counselors, librarians, nurses, food service, and so on
- School environment

Factors Outside the School

- Parents and other family members
- Cultural practices
- Religious beliefs and customs
- Social environment
- Peer influence
- Economics
- General government services
- Health and human services agencies

Each of these factors can contribute to a student's success or lack of success, but how much does each individual factor influence student performance in school? There is no valid measurement to reveal the answer. In addition, no one factor, agency, or organization can be wholly responsible for student health and social needs.

Barriers

There appear to be two main barriers to providing a comprehensive school health program for children: (1) there is no single, clear, and consistent goal for school-age children that most agencies embrace; and (2) administrators of the helping agencies and organizations often work in isolation from one another. This booklet provides techniques and processes that can be used to maximize the impact of their health programs and services.

The Goal: Collaboration

Agencies and organizations have specific reasons for existing. The Department of Health, with perhaps regional and county offices, may have many departments and divisions. One of its purposes is to provide policies (laws and rules) and services to meet the needs of school-age children and their families. Health and Human Services, also through many divisions, has as its mission to meet the needs of children and their families. The State Offices of Education have as their central purpose the education of school-age children. Although these agencies and organizations share the goal of meeting needs of children and their families, they all work independently.

The following illustration attempts to convey the expanded concept, or system, of education and services needed to effectively influence students' development and learning. This illustration suggests that the system of public school education is much larger than just the school building. The school board, administrators, and school staff do their best to help educate students during the school day. Parents, business, city and county government, social agencies, and churches also work diligently to fulfill their missions related to the health and well-being of young people.

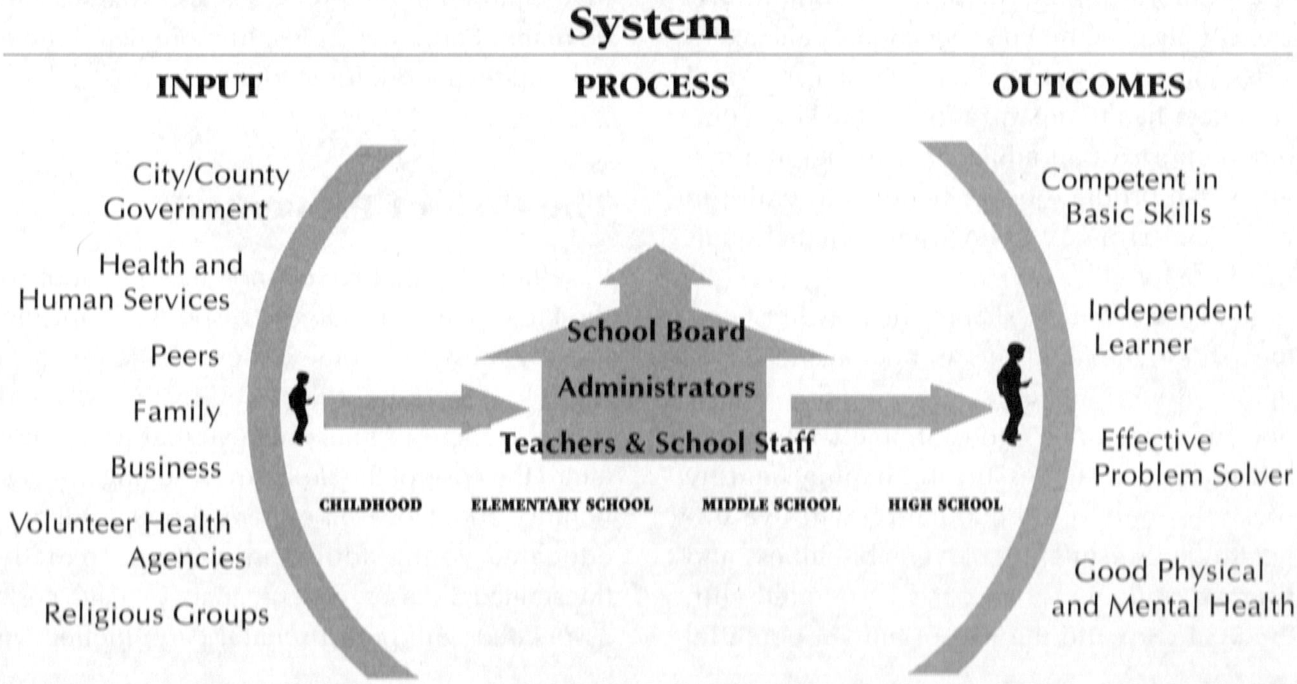

Unfortunately, education, health, and human service agencies operate independently, each one specializing in one aspect of an individual's life. Quite often they work in isolation from other helping and service organizations. Is all of this uncoordinated assistance cost-effective? If they had all pooled resources, using a comprehensive strategy, would the unhealthy conditions among adolescents and adults be as devastating as they are today? If students had adopted healthier behaviors as a result of current teaching methods, there would probably be fewer accidental deaths, fewer incidences of tobacco and other substance use, fewer cases of sexually transmitted diseases, fewer teenage mothers, fewer suicides, fewer dropouts, less antisocial behavior, and better nutritional and physical health. Missed opportunities in the past to deal with small problems have resulted in problems that have now grown so large they are almost unmanageable. Should schools, parents, and communities continue to deal with health issues among the young with the tools, techniques, and strategies of the past? If so, what is the likelihood that we will be more successful now than we were with past efforts? It's time for a new strategy.

Collaboration among parents, community, city-county government, education, health agencies, human service agencies, businesses, and volunteer health organizations is the key. Combined efforts of all adults and the helping services can produce better benefits to children with long-term cost savings and a higher quality of life for all.

To be successful in shaping healthy lifestyles, the school, the family, nonschool agencies, religious groups, and other community organizations must combine efforts. If, in the future, we are not more successful in shaping healthy lifestyles, half of the population will live unhealthy lives, suffering preventable illness and premature death. High costs associated with medical care and the loss of human potential will skyrocket. A unified, combined approach to school health will assist in positively influencing in-school and out-of-school factors that affect students' behaviors and lifestyle choices.

The educational community and parents seek the same goals for students: mastery of basic skills, independent learning, effective problem solving, and optimal physical and mental health. These goals can be met, but cooperative leadership is needed to give the system direction. Reaching the goals requires teamwork!

Building Teamwork

There is a role for everyone to play, but it must be centered on a common vision of helping students succeed. The Legislature, State Board of Education, State Education Agency and other state, regional, and local health and social organizations along with local school boards, superintendents, principals, teachers, students, parents, families, community members, and business leaders can all contribute by influencing one or more factors associated with student success and good health. If everyone works as a team, positive changes in the processes and systems can be made. Part 2 describes, in more detail, how to build teamwork for student success.

The Cost of Prevention

It is often said that we cannot afford to address the factors that are largely responsible for unhealthy lifestyles. Some believe that a person's lifestyle cannot be influenced by schools and social agencies. Others believe that we cannot afford the costs of the problems resulting from ignorance about low self-esteem, dropouts, undereducated young adults on welfare, sexually transmitted diseases, teen pregnancy, health costs associated with poor prenatal care, ineffective parenting practices, smoking, poor physical condition, malnutrition, and poor mental health. If educators examine their efforts and then look at the results, what kind of picture emerges?

The desired results of health instruction are students who will demonstrate knowledge, skills, and attitudes necessary for choosing a healthy lifestyle. A significant amount of time is spent teaching health concepts. Special programs are created, materials are purchased, lectures are given, student involvement programs are conducted, recognition and rewards are given for physical fitness, and health services are provided. A great deal of time is devoted to assessing desired results to determine the extent to which the programs and services are effective. Appraisal, assessment, evaluation, and documentation for audits, accreditation, and compliance are carried out each year. What does all of this cost? Consider the questions on this and the next page and the responses your local schools might give.

Example: Cost of Prevention vs. Remediation

1. What programs, services, or activities are carried out to monitor, assess, appraise, or audit to verify that we are getting the intended results?

Program/Activity	Estimated Costs*
• Testing: six weeks, semester end of unit	______
• Evaluation of personnel	______
• Management overhead for appraising and monitoring	______
• Low morale, follow-up and grievances	______
• Accreditation, federal compliance monitoring	______
• Record keeping, attendance monitoring, auditing	______
• Other: ______________________	______

2. If the appraisal/assessment system reveals that we have not achieved what we want, what are some of the consequences/costs of these internal and external failures?

The Internal Failures (dealt with by the school staff):

Program/Activity	Estimated Costs*
• Remediation	______
• Repeating grade/subject	______
• Discipline problems	______
• Dropouts/loss of students	______
• Other: ______________________	______

** Administrative costs for testing, compliance, dropout programs, and so on can often be obtained through your school district's accounting department.*

The External Failures (paid for by taxpayers, city, county, and state agencies):

Program/Activity	Estimated Costs#
• Dropout — marginal employment, no tax revenues, crime, prison	______
• Inability to be self-supporting, welfare	______
• Medicaid costs (inpatient hospital expenses) of births to adolescent mothers	______
• Costs of serving adolescent mothers and their children through Aid to Families with Dependent Children programs	______
• GED Program	______
• Other: ______	______

3. What can we do to prevent these failures in the system? How do their costs compare to the costs of remediation?

Preventive Measures We Can Take:	Estimated Costs**
• Parenting/family counseling	______
• Early childhood — 3- to 4-year-old program	______
• Effective dropout prevention programs	______
• Staff development and training for committees	______
• School-to-work transition	______
• School-based services, collaboration with other agencies	______
• Comprehensive health education	______
• Tutoring and summer schools	______
• More community and parental support for high academic performances	______
• Other: ______	______

 # Cost estimates for prison costs, welfare spending, Medicaid, and Aid to Families with Dependent Children (AFDC) programs can often be obtained through state Departments of Health and Human Services and State Departments of Justice. For example, in 1988, the U.S. taxpayers spent nearly $20 billion to support families that began with a birth to an adolescent mother. This total includes AFDC, Medicaid and Food Stamps. The Center for Population Options estimates the United States would have saved $8 billion if every birth to an adolescent mother had been delayed (4).

***Administrative costs for tutoring, staff-development training, and dropout prevention programs can often be obtained through your district's accounting department.*

In most cases, it becomes evident that it costs a great deal more to fix problems than to prevent them. In addition, the cost of fixing problems does not take into account the human costs suffered by those who do poorly academically, socially, and economically.

Adding more assessment and evaluation will not address the challenges unless fundamental changes in the system are made. One change can be the way in which agencies cooperate to achieve the same goals for students. Another way to begin the change is to examine the way in which data are used to design or redesign programs and services.

What Are the Health Facts in Your Community?

The health issues facing society as a whole also influence the health and well-being of individuals in your community. What are the health facts in your community? How effective have your school health programs been in addressing student health needs? Using the questions listed in the chart that follows, estimate the major health issues among school-age children in your county, city, or school district. These figures can be obtained from your local school district, law enforcement agency, and health departments. Many statistics, such as the incidence of sexual activity and of tobacco and other drug use, are difficult to measure but can be estimated based on the following:

Health-Related Issues	National *	Your State	Your Community
• How many youth in secondary schools have used alcohol, tobacco, inhalants, and/or illicit drugs in the past 30 days?	Thirty-six percent of 11,631 high school students surveyed report using tobacco, while 14 percent report using marijuana within 30 days of completing the questionnaire. Thirty-seven percent had five or more drinks on one occasion (7). It is estimated that over 3.5 million 12- to 17-year-olds have tried marijuana (8).		
• How many youth under the age of 18 have no medical insurance?	Estimates indicate that 15 percent of adolescents (4.7 million) have no medical insurance (4).		
• How many reported cases of sexually transmitted disease (STD) occur in youth under the age of 20?	The Centers for Disease Control and Prevention (CDC) estimates that approximately 2.5 million adolescents contract an STD each year. Thousands are infected with HIV, with AIDS being one of the ten leading causes of deaths in adolescents. By the end of 1992, there were 10,528 cases of AIDS among young people under the age of 25 reported to the CDC. Between December 1990 and December 1992, the number of AIDS cases among 13- to 24-year-olds increased by 43 percent (10). These numbers do not take into account the numerous undiagnosed cases of chlamydia and pelvic inflammatory diseases.		

Health Facts *continued*

Health-Related Issues	National *	Your State	Your Community
• How many babies were born to girls ages 15-19?	More than 1 million (1 in 10) teenagers get pregnant every year. Current estimates indicate that over 2,700 American teenagers become pregnant every day (7). The birth rate among unmarried adolescents under the age of 20 has increased 300 percent for whites and 16 percent for blacks (4). An American teenager has a baby approximately every 61 seconds (517,635 in 1992) (9).		
• How many youth have trouble with the law because of alcohol or other drugs?	Every 7 minutes an American youth is arrested for a drug offense (approximately 76,986 per year), while every 30 minutes an American youth is arrested for drunken driving (approximately 17,674 per year) (11).		
• What percentage of students drop out before completing high school?	Approximately 30 percent of American high school students drop out each year (12).		
• How many youth are victims of violence (family, outside, or self-inflicted)?	Every year over 2 million children and adolescents are reported abused or neglected. The suicide rate for teenagers has doubled since 1968, making it the second leading cause of death among adolescents. Among 15- to 19-year-old minority youth, homicide is the leading cause of death (8).		

** See Data Source in Bibliography*

Regardless of how you organize to address health needs, student and staff well-being must be a priority for schools. A look at the *facts* about health conditions among the school-age children in your area, and an awareness of the powerful role staff plays in modeling and shaping healthy behaviors in students, will help guide your efforts.

Building an Approach

If your school chooses to address one or more health issue(s) believed important for student success and well-being, you must consider addressing such issues in a comprehensive way. As the team forms its concept for a coordinated system that works, consider what researchers in the field of comprehensive school health programming say: Classroom health instruction and health services are only two aspects of a comprehensive school health program.

The informal survey provided on the following page is based on the expanded concept of comprehensive school health first suggested by Diane Allensworth and Lloyd Kolbe (5). The survey is divided into the eight components of a comprehensive school health program: health instruction, health services, school environment, counseling and guidance, physical education, school food service, parent/community involvement for healthy schools, and employee health promotions. Everyone who is involved in the school health improvement team should read the questions and check one of the three responses (satisfied, somewhat satisfied, or dissatisfied) that best reflects his or her perceptions. Opportunities should be provided to the team members to ask questions. After everyone has completed the survey, a group member should collect all the responses and compile a summary. The sample summary sheet provided following the survey (see pages 13-14) will assist in organizing the discussion.

Part 2 of this booklet will guide you through a more in-depth survey of needs. The purpose of this initial informal survey is to raise the group's level of awareness as well as to assess individuals' perceptions of needs. Because this informal survey is requesting the level of *satisfaction* with the current program, there are no right or wrong answers.

COMPREHENSIVE SCHOOL HEALTH—INFORMAL SURVEY

What are the major health problems facing children and youth in your community?

☐ **Accidents**
☐ **Suicide**
☐ **School-age pregnancy**
☐ **Poor nutrition**
☐ **HIV or other sexually transmitted diseases**
☐ **Tobacco use**
☐ **Drug and alcohol use**
☐ **Poor physical fitness**
☐ **Abuse and neglect**
☐ **Violence and gangs**
☐ **Environmental hazards**
☐ **Other**

Are you satisfied with your school health programs?
Check the response that best reflects your thoughts.

Dissatisfied | Somewhat Satisfied | Satisfied

Are you satisfied with your school's health instruction program?
Does it teach skills and healthy behaviors or just provide information? Are students knowledgeable about health issues and facts? Are they skilled in using this knowledge to make decisions about their health? Does the program include teaching and learning about consumer health, community health, environmental health, family life and reproductive health, growth and development, nutritional health, personal health, prevention and control of disease, safety and accident prevention, and substance use and abuse? Does the curriculum address intellectual and emotional as well as physical health? Is it designed to motivate students not only to prevent disease but also to live healthier lives?

Are you satisfied with your school's health services?
Are immunization standards met, appropriate screenings completed, and referrals made efficiently? Is your school's health care worker a resource for parents,teachers, health educators, counselors, and staff? Do your school health services help students and staff become healthier or just tend to their immediate physical health needs?

Are you satisfied with your school's environment?
Are both the social *and* physical environments conducive to teaching and learning? Do your district's goals for students and your school's policies and administrative behavior encourage a businesslike, friendly, open, and caring environment? Are your school's facilities clean, safe, and orderly? Do the air, water, and buildings put students at physical risk, or do they help students learn?

Are you satisfied with your school's counseling and guidance services?
Are the services part of an integrated effort involving parents, teachers, and administrators? Do they include individual and group counseling, career counseling, peer assistance, assessments, and intervention programs? Are there programs for learning life skills, problem solving, substance abuse prevention, and self-esteem? Do the programs help improve student behavior, reduce drug use, increase student/staff cooperation and make students feel good about themselves and school?

Are you satisfied with your school's physical education program?
Does it help students develop and maintain cardio-respiratory efficiency, muscular strength, endurance and flexibility? Does it encourage the development of lifetime leisure skills? Do team sports, band, choir, or other extra-curricular activities supplement daily physical activity, or do they just replace it? Do students meet the standards appropriate to their grade level?

Are you satisfied with your school's food services?
Do they serve nutritious meals that the students like? Do your food services strive to follow the USDA guidelines for good nutrition? Is there education for both students and staff about good nutrition? Do your school's snack and drink machines offer healthy choices?

Are you satisfied with parent and community involvement in health promotion efforts?
Does your community have a health council made up of classroom teachers; support staff; administrators; parents; businesses; state, county, and local governments; and volunteer health organizations? Has your community effectively developed the plans necessary to change policy and focus attention on school health issues? Are there cost-effective programs that help reduce or eliminate health problems? Is most of the community satisfied that efforts are unified and results achieved?

Are you satisfied with your school's employee health promotion programs?
Do you have programs that promote employee wellness? Are your staff members healthy role models for the students? Are you satisfied with your school's productivity? Are you satisfied with the amount of money spent on health insurance claims and absenteeism?

Call to Action: If you checked "dissatisfied" in two or more areas, it's time to take a closer look at your school health programs.

Sample Summary Sheet

	Dissatisfied	Somewhat Satisfied	Satisfied
1. Are you satisfied with your school's health-instruction program?	☐	☐	☐
Comments:			
2. Are you satisfied with your school's health services?	☐	☐	☐
Comments:			
3. Are you satisfied with your school's environment?	☐	☐	☐
Comments:			
4. Are you satisfied with your school's counseling and guidance services?	☐	☐	☐
Comments:			
5. Are you satisfied with your school's physical education program?	☐	☐	☐
Comments:			

Sample Summary Sheet *continued*

	Dissatisfied	Somewhat Satisfied	Satisfied
6. Are you satisfied with your school's food service program?	☐	☐	☐
Comments:			
7. Are you satisfied with your school's parent/community involvement?	☐	☐	☐
Comments:			
8. Are you satisfied with your school's employee health promotion program?	☐	☐	☐
Comments:			

Once the tally has been totaled, it is usually helpful to discuss the results to clarify the meaning of responses and comments.

Summary and Next Steps

Many factors contribute to the success of students. Teamwork and combined resources are essential to effectively address all the factors that shape and influence student behaviors and lifestyles.

What, then, is the vision that the school board, school staff, parents, community members, and business leaders can share regarding effective school health programs? Discuss your hopes and expectations for comprehensive school health with other members of the group. Write down the key elements of the vision and then use it as a reference point for site-based decision making and planning. In Part 2, there are some specific activities that can help you formulate and shape a vision for your school.

Getting Started

Get the facts about health conditions and programs to serve students and adults in your community. Here are some ways to get the facts and assess needs:

- Calculate the cost of prevention versus remediation using the guidelines provided on pages 7–8 of this booklet and share this information with the School Board, the site-based decision-making committee, parents, and other community members. Seek communitywide acceptance of shared responsibility for meeting student needs, and seek cooperation among all agencies and organizations that help students and their families.
- Get the facts about the health conditions of youth in your community and programs available (pages 9–10) — both school services and out-of-school services (for example: what health education curriculum is used, when health instruction is provided, what nursing services are provided, and so on). Involve the committee in discussing the facts in your community.
- Prioritize your needs. Using the health findings in your community and the results of individuals' perceived level of satisfaction (see informal survey, page 12), prioritize areas for action (health services, health curriculum, community outreach, employee health promotion, and so on). Remember, not all priorities can be addressed at once. The challenge to the group is to build consensus and, initially, to select one or two areas for action. The more comprehensive survey in Appendix A will assist the group in selecting areas for action.
- Design a site-based plan to increase prevention efforts and to reduce costly remediation programs. Programs must cut across the traditional boundaries of disciplines and professions. Gain commitment from parents, community members, business and industry, and helping agencies to work cooperatively to overcome the barriers of turf protection, fragmented programs, categorical programs, and traditional roles.
- Focus attention on results. Reduce blame and seek to address the causes of problems. Seek to determine the cause-and-effect relationships between programs and desired results.

Children are indeed the future. Their education and health must be of the utmost concern to everyone. Only when children are achieving at the peak of their abilities can they be prepared to lead the nation in the twenty-first century. Together, families, schools, the health community, and the public and private sectors must forge partnerships to meet the interrelated health and education needs of our children. Through effective collaboration, we can provide young people with the tools to become healthy, productive adults.

Part 2

Planning a Comprehensive School Health Program

Introduction

As discussed in Part 1 and reflected in the following illustration, the "system" to help students achieve the goals set for them is much larger than just the school building. Students spend a great deal of time away from school with their peers and families and in the community.

Quite often education, as well as the social services system, is organized to act independently when trying to meet needs. In the face of the immediate challenges, it is imperative to mobilize all resources and make a coordinated effort to ensure that today's children become tomorrow's healthy, productive adults and parents.

Site-Based Decision Making and A Vision

Schools may have site-based decision-making (SBDM) committees that discuss the needs of their students in order to establish campus performance objectives, develop long-range plans, and provide input into curriculum, budgeting,

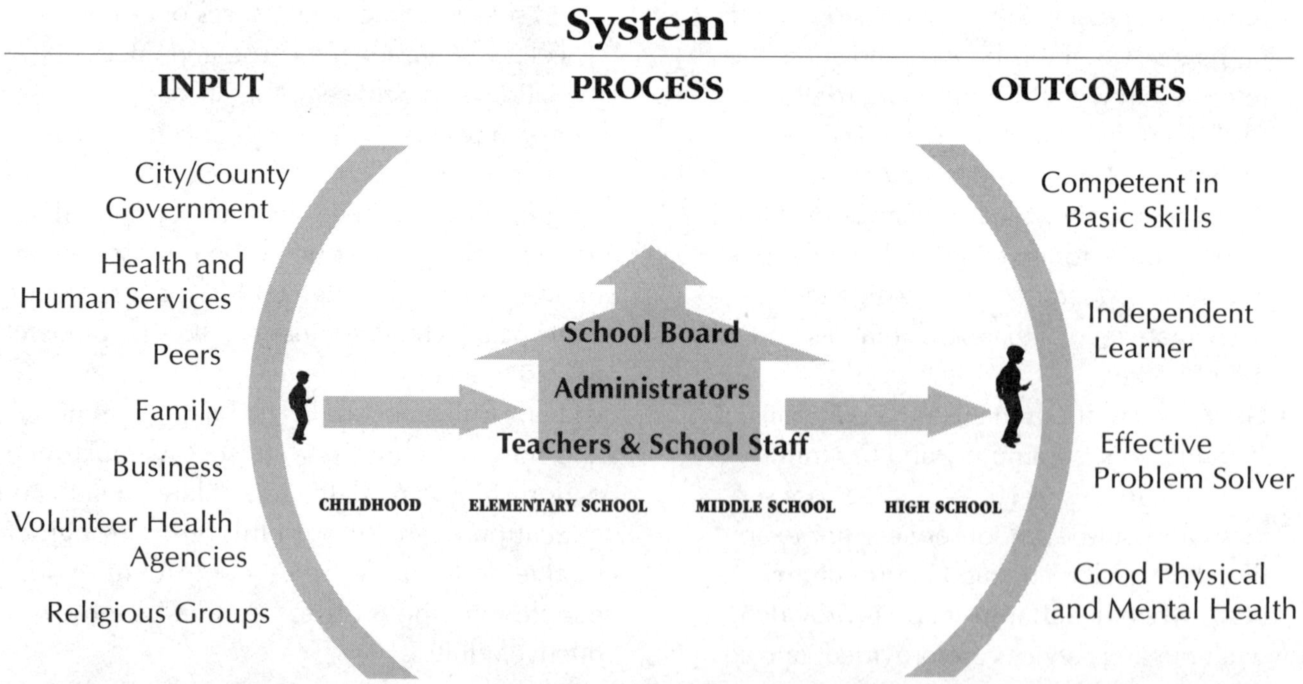

staffing patterns, and school organization. One role of such committees is to priortize the goals so that energy and resources can be focused on meeting expectations set by the group. However, without a clear sense of direction and consensus on the desired results, it will be difficult for committee members to work together as a team. Teamwork is created by developing a common vision of the conditions committee members would like to bring about in their school.

The vision to guide individual schools in achieving desired results for their students must be developed locally so that it reflects the parents' and community's aspirations for their students. The vision will no doubt address the physical, mental/emotional, and social health of students. The next section outlines a process that will help guide your team in developing its vision.

Developing a Shared Vision

Almost everyone will agree that if you don't have a clear picture of where you are going, you may end up someplace else. Currently, most school efforts are driven by a combination of external forces, internal forces, and inertia. There may be, in many cases, no vision.

Sometimes plans are made in response to state mandates and programs and services of the past, with very little examination of their appropriateness, adequacy, or effectiveness. In a shared vision for your school, such issues are addressed. The broader the base of involvement, the more likely the vision will be supported, pursued, and realized.

In preparing to develop or clarify the vision for school health, the entire system of public school education must be considered. Health concerns must be addressed within the context of school life, community life, and family life. The SBDM team or the school health council should include:

- parents.
- community members.
- business representatives.
- teachers, counselors, nurses, and other school staff.
- representatives of religious groups.
- state, county, or local health agency representatives.
- human services representatives.
- representatives of volunteer health organizations.

A broad-based representative group is suggested as ad hoc members, because they are part of the system of helping students achieve the desired exit-level skills resulting from elementary and secondary education. It is important that they also have a sense of ownership and commitment to the expectations for students.

In developing a vision statement the group can consider these questions: What programs would best serve the needs of students? What conditions must exist in the school, in the community, among family members, and among state, county, city service providers and other helping agencies? What would the ideal system and process look like? The vision statement can include both a vision of the process and a vision of the desired results. It requires the group's commitment and teamwork.

The following is an example of a vision statement:

In the ________________ community, school staff, parents, school board members, community members, health and human service agencies, and volunteer health organizations work together in planning and implementing health promotion programs for students and staff. Through this cooperation, programs and services are successful in encouraging healthy lifestyles among students and staff, and in reducing preventable diseases and premature deaths.

Each community must develop its own unique vision. The site-based decision-making team or school health council should take the time to discuss and describe what ideal conditions everyone would like to see. Summarize the thoughts and ideas into a brief statement that everyone can support.

In the process of developing a vision statement, it is vital that the school board and other chief school policy makers support the group's efforts. This is the only way to gain approval for policies spelling out the particulars for the comprehensive school health program and for program implementation. Although the vision may be clear, the steps toward reaching that vision must be tailored to take advantage of the programs already in place or available within each school and community. Once a shared vision is developed, program goals, or desired results for students, are needed to further guide efforts.

Desired Results for Students

Many school districts already have goals for student learning, a mission statement, and other written forms stating their expectations of all students by the time they exit high school. But, who "owns" these goals? What level of commitment exists to pursue the goals? How often are they used as a real framework to assess progress? Are they representative of the diversity of interest within the community? Do the goals take into consideration the students' physical and mental well-being? The challenge lies not so much in developing a set of desired results for students, but rather in developing a sense of ownership and commitment among all concerned in achieving these goals.

It is beyond the scope of this booklet to describe in detail the variety of approaches that can be used to develop commitment to desired results for students and for public schools. However, commitment is clearly a prerequisite to developing a unified, well-supported plan for all students. Any method that offers a structure to the discussion and debate concerning the desired behaviors of schoolchildren will work among people of goodwill. For purposes of illustration, the following is one way desired exit behaviors could be stated:

SAMPLE SCHOOL

Desired Exit Behaviors for Students

By the time students exit the SAMPLE school, each will demonstrate that he or she:

- is self-directed as a learner and an individual.
- has high self-esteem as a learner and an individual.
- is able to solve problems, make decisions, and understand cause-effect relationships.
- has concern for others and the environment.
- accepts responsibility for his or her own physical and mental well-being.
- has academic skills essential to being a productive member of society.

In order to ensure that students acquire these skills, the school will direct efforts in all subjects and disciplines to achieve these desired results for all students. As decisions are made at the classroom, campus, and district levels, they will be tested against this question: To what extent will this decision help us achieve one or more of these desired results?

Identifying Desired Results

Once desired exit behaviors for students are defined, the group can identify those behaviors or desired characteristics central to the student's well-being. You will probably find that most desired exit-level behaviors for students combine cognitive development with physical and emotional development.

Mastery of basic skills, high self-esteem, and good physical and mental health are all required in order for a student to be an effective self-directed learner, problem solver, and decision maker. English language arts, mathematics, social studies, and health education can focus on these ultimate desired results for student development as well. If the primary concern is a healthy, productive child, everyone can work together to make student *growth,* as opposed to mastery of a single subject, the goal. The student and the community will benefit from this collaborative approach to addressing the needs of the whole child.

Assessing Current Conditions

Once your vision statement and exit-level behaviors are established, it is time to analyze programs and services currently in place to achieve the desired results. Part 1 included an informal survey to assess your group's level of satisfaction with the current school health programs and services. The informal survey raises the awareness of comprehensive school health. The survey provided in Appendix A offers a more in-depth look at your programs. Some members may be pleasantly surprised to find that many programs and services are already working cooperatively. However, other members may be equally surprised to find that the system is not working well for many students. Improvement may be needed.

Completing the Comprehensive School Health Survey

The Comprehensive School Health (CSH) Survey, along with survey instructions, is provided in Appendix A on page 28. You will notice that, as in the informal survey in Part 1, school health has been divided into eight components: health instruction, health services, school environment, counseling and guidance, physical education, food service, parent/community involvement and employee health promotion. Opportunities should be provided to the team to ask questions. After everyone has completed the survey, a group member should collect all the responses and compile a summary. Summary findings are then plotted on the circular graph provided on page 40 at the end of the survey.

Selecting Areas for Action

Completing the CSH Survey and plotting the findings on the circular graph will provide the group with a "snapshot" of the level of perceived effectiveness in eight areas related to school health programming. Those areas that rated an average of 1.5 or less out of 3 may be the areas your group selects for priority attention. For example, perhaps the group indicated that many of the statements related to health instruction were "not descriptive" or only "somewhat descriptive" of their current school's/district's health instruction program, giving an average rating of 1.5 on a scale of 3. The health instruction program may then become the group's focus for improvement. Keep in mind that the selection of a priority does not mean that work should not be done in other areas; it means that the group will focus on the *priority* until conditions are improved.

Summary and Next Steps

The above information outlines the procedure for developing a shared vision, assessing needs, and setting priorities. The next task for the group is to study the problems and to develop a plan of action. Part 3 will guide you through the process of identifying major problems in the system of delivering effective school health programs. It will help you specify the probable cause of identified problems, and develop a plan of action to address the specific factors that prevent the system from working well. Each committee member has a critical voice in developing the vision and plan whose goal is developing healthy students.

Part 3

Implementing a Comprehensive School Health Program

Introduction

Your committee is now well on its way to building healthy schools through effective school health programs. As emphasized earlier, collaboration with parents and other groups and organizations, along with coordination of services, is the key to success.

Part 1 identified the need for comprehensive school health, discussed the cost of prevention versus treatment, and provided an overview of the elements of a comprehensive school health program. Part 2 discussed developing a shared vision, offered tools for assessing your school's/community's programs, and suggested ways to select priority areas for action.

Part 3 will assist your group in identifying the factors and probable causes of failures in the system. It will also help you develop strategies to meet identified needs and evaluate program success in meeting desired student results. Ultimately, success is measured by the extent to which all children develop into healthy, self-directed young adults who are prepared to be contributing members of families, communities, and society as a whole.

Taking Action

Review the areas of need reflected in your responses on page 40 to the CSH Survey provided in Appendix A. Consider the factors or problems that led the group to identify a particular area for action. Review the findings of your committee's survey. Using the example given in Part 2, suppose your group decides to focus on improving the health instruction program. Before a plan for improvement can be developed, your committee must consider the following: What are the specific problems related to the current school health instruction program? What aspects of the instruction program caused the group ratings to be low?

The committee may want to conduct a brainstorming session when answering these questions. In that way all committee members have an opportunity to share their ideas. Since your group represents a variety of interests, it is important to obtain the various points of view and experiences that such a diverse group will bring to the discussion.

Prior to such a session, participants must be provided with an overview of the curriculum instructional methods currently in place.

When everyone understands the current instructional process, a brainstorming session to discuss problems in the system can begin. The following section provides one method for conducting such a session.

Brainstorming Major Problems

Here are some suggested steps for brainstorming the major problems as the committee perceives them. In *italics* under the steps is an example of how a brainstorming session might be used in the hypothetical situation noted above (problems with the school health instruction program).

1. Frame the focus question or issue so that it has group support.
   Focus Question: What are the major problems with the current health instruction program that prevent students from acquiring the basic health knowledge, attitude, and skills necessary for adopting healthy lifestyle choices?

2. Allow a few minutes for each member to jot down one or two ideas on index cards or gum-backed note paper.

3. Go around the table, asking each group member to state one idea regarding the issue. Then have each individual post the gum-backed paper or note card onto a flip chart at the front of the room. Posting notes rather than recording individual statements saves time as well as ensures the individual's thoughts are in his or her own words. During this stage of brainstorming, there should be no questions, comments, discussion, or interruptions. Circle the table twice, and then ask if anyone would like to add an idea not already stated. Going around the room in this fashion encourages everyone to participate, but an individual should be free to "pass."

Rather than suggesting a modification to someone else's statement, add a new one even if it seems to be quite similar.

Brainstorming ideas may generate a list such as the following:

- *The health curriculum is incomplete/ outdated.*
- *Health instruction is not a priority with the district (i.e., no clear policies or resources are provided for purchasing of materials, training, or hiring a teacher with specialization in health).*
- *Health is not an integral part of the curriculum. At the elementary level, topics are taught by teachers who are interested and take the time to acquire teaching materials. At the secondary level, less than one year of health is provided. Health issues are generally covered in a one-shot assembly session (i.e., not enough time is devoted to teaching health).*
- *At the secondary level, no individual is trained in the area. Health is taught by a coach whose focus is on athletic achievement rather than comprehensive school health instruction (i.e., staff member assigned to teach health at the secondary level does not have the interest, confidence, or competence to educate students about the vast array of issues related to healthy bodies and healthy choices).*
- *Staff development and training are not provided in current health issues and teaching techniques.*

After all group members have had an opportunity to share all their ideas, the group can rank the major concerns. The top two or three issues can become candidates for priority action. Using the list of concerns expressed during the brainstorming session, each person is asked to rate the statements as they affect the health instruction curriculum.

The ratings are as follows:

3 — if seen as a critical problem
2 — if seen as a moderately important problem
1 — if seen as a minor problem

Each member's rating should be recorded on the flip chart. When everyone has rated the items, calculate the totals for each one. Create a bar chart with the highest priority on top, and record the number of points assigned by the group. For example, if 10 individuals rated each item, the maximum number of points that any one issue could obtain is 30 (10 people all rating the same item 3, or critical). Here is an example of a chart that might have been developed from the ranking process.

Ranking Areas of Concern Related to the Health Instruction Program

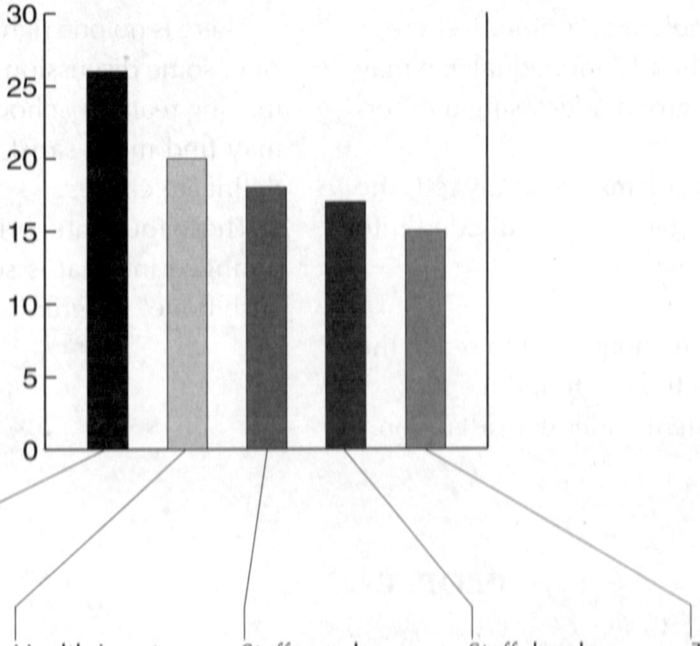

Health instruction is not a priority with the district (no clear policies or resources are provided). **26**

Health is not an integral part of the curriculum. **20**

Staff member assigned to teach health at the secondary level does not have the interest, confidence, or competence to educate students about the vast array of issues related to healthy bodies and healthy choices. **18**

Staff development and training are not provided in current health issues and teaching techniques. **17**

The health curriculum is incomplete and outdated. **15**

Understanding Causes and Effects

Through the use of the needs-assessment instruments in Parts 1 and 2, your group has now identified a specific area of action to target for improvement (the health instruction program in our example). Using the brainstorming technique in Part 3 allowed you to rank underlying problems, such as the health instruction program's not being a priority in the district. The group is now ready to target the causes of the problems to be addressed through collaborative efforts. Make sure the causes reflect specific factors that prevent the system from working well. To do this, address one problem at a time. If there is a large group (more than 10 individuals), it may be subdivided, each group addressing a different problem.

When complex problems are analyzed, the probable causes can generally be divided into the following four categories.

Methods: The methods used to reach the objectives or to reduce the problem under consideration.

Materials: The materials used in the processes of teaching, learning, and in the diagnosis and treatment of illnesses.

People: Factors associated with people involved in one or more of the entities seeking to reach the same outcome or goal.

Policies: The state/city/county school policies that are aimed at helping children and supporting the attainment of the long-term goal of healthy and productive young adults.

There is no one right way to categorize causes. After some discussion, your site-based decision-making team or school health advisory council may find more satisfactory ways to group and delineate causes.

These four categories of probable causes are arranged in what is sometimes referred to as a "fish bone" diagram, as illustrated below:

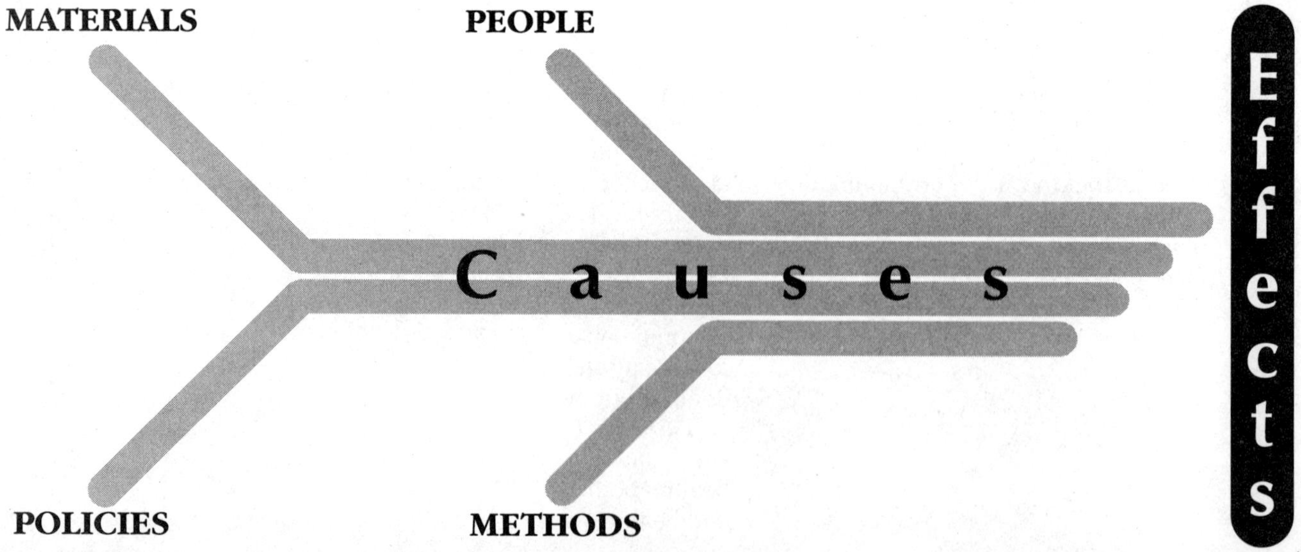

State a problem the group has identified as critical to achieving the overall desired outcome. Discuss how the outcome can be measured so that the effectiveness of actions taken can be evaluated. For example, students leaving the fifth grade should have adequate, age-appropriate knowledge of health issues related to healthy bodies and healthy choices. Attitude, behavior, and knowledge of such health issues can be measured by a sixth-grade basic skills test and attitude and behavior survey. For those students entering the middle grades who have not reached the expected results, we must ask: what are the major causes/underlying factors? A cause-and-effect diagram may look like the one at the bottom of this page.

Categorizing causes of problems associated with school health programs and services allows the committee to then develop an action plan to remedy the underlying causes of "system failure."

Action for Program Improvement

Your group has now identified the perceived areas of needs concerning school health, brainstormed the problems in the current system, and categorized the underlying causes of the problems into one or more of the following areas: methods, materials, people, and/or policies.

Your action plan should be built upon goals, objectives, and strategies to address the probable cause. For example, again using the hypothetical situation above, the problem may be stated like this: School health instruction is not a priority and suffers from inadequate policy support. The goals and objectives may focus on increasing policy support. The action plan may include strategies such as presentations to the school board that highlight the need for CSH programming, awareness sessions to parent groups and other community members, or articles published in the local newspaper. Appendix B on page 41 provides a sample action plan form.

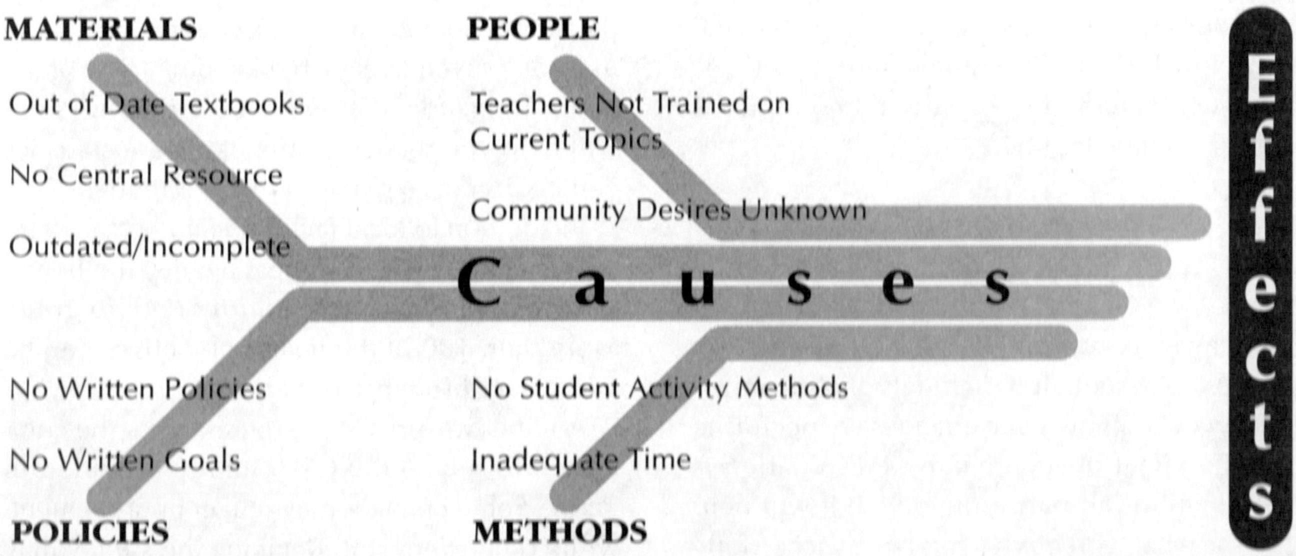

Working Your Plan

The action plan that the committee outlined provides the starting point and the subsequent steps that need to be taken. A task may require the work of one individual or several committee members. Tasks must be doable and time lines must be realistic.

Numerous agencies and organizations have materials to assist you in your efforts. Appendix E on page 50 is a resource directory of state and national organizations that provide resources and support for addressing a variety of health and education issues.

Tapping into local resources is essential to working your plan. It is important to involve local health agencies, parents, churches, youth groups and other organizations. By enlisting local groups and individuals, the committee is establishing grassroots support. Community involvement provides the resources and support needed to reduce fragmentation of efforts or duplication of programs. Ongoing collaboration and cooperation between the team and other community members also prevents unwarranted controversy that may arise as a result of poor communication or collaboration.

Ensuring the continued support by agencies and individuals will be easier if there is feedback on the status of each task. Communication and coordination of each task is essential to the accomplishment of the goals and objectives. Tasks will need to be reassessed and reprioritized from time to time.

Measuring Progress

Assessment, or measurement, of the committee's progress is essential. Individuals and organizations want to know what changes are occurring and the effect of such changes. Evaluation is beneficial for all parties involved. It will help identify what works, what has been successfully changed, and where the community is in this process of change.

Assessment of the committee's progress can be charted by noting completion of each task on the action plan. This step allows the committee to identify what has been done and what tasks remain incomplete or need to be broken down into smaller tasks and reassigned. The group must ask: If we accomplish the tasks we've set out to do, what positive differences will be made for our students, ourselves, and our community?

The status of your school's progress toward implementing a comprehensive school health program can be assessed by comparing your school health program against a set of voluntary guidelines or standards for comprehensive school health provided in Appendix C on page 42. These standards are intended to assist rather than to judge schools. Stated in broad terms, the standards are descriptive rather than prescriptive. They state what the intended desired results are, but do not prescribe how to get there. Thus the standards allow each school and community to build a comprehensive school health program in a manner that best fits the needs of the community.

Program success can also be assessed by reviewing the health statistics in your community. Statistically significant changes in the health indicators of your community's children and youth may take several years, but keeping track of the major indicators that were identified in Part 1 will help you recognize trends. These statistics can be used as a guide for the committee.

In addition to local facts and figures, the committee can measure progress against the health objectives outlined in *Healthy People 2000.* More than 100 of the health objectives can be addressed through school health programs.

Another way to assess progress is for the committee to retake the CSH Survey provided in Part 2. Some changes may reflect improvement, while others may not. Retaking the survey may be beneficial for adjusting the action plan. This procedure allows for changes to accommodate new information or new factors that are important to the success of the action plan.

Not all changes may be reflected when retaking the CSH Survey. Therefore, anecdotal reports will prove useful in measuring progress. Individuals may have heard of some factor or change that had a positive effect on students, teachers, parents, or other community members. For example, an employee health promotion program may increase employee morale long before the improvement can be measured in a reduced number of sick days. Likewise, a school-linked health care program may improve school/community relations and access to care before it is reflected in improved attendance. Although anecdotal reports may not initially reflect quantifiable desired results, they provide important considerations when dealing with school health programs.

In addition to program desired results, the committee *process* should also be evaluated. Appendix D on page 49 provides a sample report for evaluating the committee's accomplishments, morale and relationships, and operations.

However the committee decides to measure its progress, the important concept to consider is the vision statement. The vision statement should continue to guide all work of the committee.

Summary

Promoting a Comprehensive School Health Program has been developed to assist schools and communities in focusing on the goal of a healthy future for all children. The assessment instruments, comprehensive school health standards, and resource directory are intended to help local communities and school committees and councils in this quest.

Part 1 is designed to increase individual and community understanding of what comprehensive school health is, and to demonstrate the need for comprehensive school-health programming. Part 2 provides tools to facilitate assessing local needs and setting priorities for action. Part 3 contains a framework for planning strategies to address local needs and priorities. The Appendixes include additional tools: a comprehensive school health survey, a sample action planning form, a set of voluntary standards (guidelines) for comprehensive school health programs, a checklist to evaluate the workings of the school health advisory council, and a resource directory of national public, private, and nonprofit health and education agencies and organizations.

Everyone must be committed to supporting a healthy future by encouraging local schools, parents, and communities to address the interrelated health and education needs of children and youth. This resource will assist you in your efforts. Together, educators, parents, and community members can create a healthy, thriving learning environment where all schoolchildren have every opportunity to enter adulthood as productive, participating members of society.

Appendix A

Comprehensive School Health Survey

General Instructions

After receiving an orientation concerning comprehensive school health (CSH) and the eight areas of a CSH program (health instruction, health services, school environment, counseling and guidance, physical education, food service, parent/community involvement, and employee health promotion), each individual should complete the *Comprehensive School Health Survey* on the following pages. The survey is divided into the eight areas of a CSH program, with eight questions per CSH area. Complete as many items as possible. Your *perceptions* are most important, so you do not need to be an expert in any of the eight areas of CSH.

Step 1:

- Read each of the statements describing elements of a CSH program. There are 8 statements for each of the 8 areas, for a total of 64 statements.

- Place a ✔ under one of the three columns on the *Comprehensive School Health Survey* to indicate the extent to which you believe each statement is descriptive of your district or campus. The three choices are as follows: Not Descriptive, Somewhat Descriptive, or Very Descriptive.

Step 2:

- After responding to the 64 statements by placing a ✔ in the appropriate column, you will give each of the 8 areas (instruction, services, environment, counseling and guidance, physical education, food service, parent/community involvement, and employee health promotion) a numerical rating.

- For each of the items checked, assign a numerical rating using the following scale:

Not Descriptive	=	1 point
Somewhat Descriptive	=	2 points
Very Descriptive	=	3 points

- Add the scores from each column to get a total score for each of the 8 areas of CSH. For example, if you checked "Very Descriptive" for all 8 statements in the health instruction section, the total score for health instruction would be 24 (8 statements x 3 points per statement).

- Transfer the total scores for each of the 8 areas onto the *Individual Summary Sheet.*

Step 3:

- Collect all the individual summary sheets and record individual total scores on the *Group Summary Sheet.*

- Calculate the sum of all scores for each of the 8 areas of CSH and enter in the column labeled "Sum" on the *Group Summary Sheet.*

- Divide the summary scores by the number of individuals completing the survey and place this number in the column labeled "Average Score" on the *Group Summary Sheet.* This will give you an overall average total score for each of the 8 areas of CSH.

- Divide the average total score by 8 (the number of statements in each of the 8 areas of CSH), and place this number in the column labeled "Average Rating" on the *Group Summary Sheet.* This will give you an average rating for all items within the 8 areas of CSH.

  For example: If 4 people completed the survey and all 4 individuals checked "Very Descriptive" for all 8 statements within the health instruction area, you would have the following:

  Total for Health Instruction for Each Person . . . . 24 (3 pts. x 8 items)
  Sum of all Scores for Health Instruction . . . . 96 (24 total pts. x 4 respondents)
  Average Score for Health Instruction . . . . 24 (96 sum ÷ 4 respondents)
  Average Rating for All Statements Within Health . . . . 3 (24 total ÷ 8 statements)

Step 4:

- Transfer the average rating scores for each of the 8 areas to the *Comprehensive School Health Profile* (the circular graph). This will provide a "snapshot" of your current CSH program as seen by individuals completing the survey.

- When working in program improvement, your group may want to focus on those items rated 1.5 or lower (closer to the center of the circular graph).

Comprehensive School Health Survey

HEALTH INSTRUCTION

STEP 1

To what extent do the following statements characterize your school/district?

	Not Descriptive	Somewhat Descriptive	Very Descriptive
1. The health curriculum content is balanced among the ten content areas: community health, consumer health, environmental health, family life, growth and development, nutritional health, personal health, prevention and control of disease, safety and accident prevention, and substance use and abuse.	❑	❑	❑
2. The health instruction program provides activities to develop decision-making skills related to health and encourages wellness, instead of merely disease prevention.	❑	❑	❑
3. Health instruction exceeds the minimum state requirements.	❑	❑	❑
4. Appropriate and effective health instructional materials are available, and training is provided in the use of instructional materials.	❑	❑	❑
5. Ongoing staff development and in-service training in current health issues and teaching techniques are provided.	❑	❑	❑
6. There are clear school/district goals and objectives for health instruction stated in terms of specific student results expected at each grade level.	❑	❑	❑
7. Formative and summative evaluations are used to appropriately measure student knowledge, attitudes, and behaviors related to health.	❑	❑	❑
8. Parents, community members, and business representatives are satisfied with the quality and adequacy of the school's/district's health instruction.	❑	❑	❑
	(1 pt. each ✔)	(2 pts. each ✔)	(3 pts. each ✔)

COMMENTS:

_________ + _________ + _________ =
Total Column 1 Total Column 2 Total Column 3

____
Total Score

Comprehensive School Health Survey

HEALTH SERVICES

To what extent do the following statements characterize your school/district?

	Not Descriptive	Somewhat Descriptive	Very Descriptive
1. The school/district has clearly written and defined goals relating to school health.	❑	❑	❑
2. An adequate amount of staff time and personnel is allotted to screening, surveillance, and management of health problems.	❑	❑	❑
3. Referral, coordination, and collaboration with other school staff members and professional agencies are employed in the delivery of health services.	❑	❑	❑
4. Referral, coordination, and collaboration exist among health and human service and volunteer health organizations (cancer, heart, lung, and so on).	❑	❑	❑
5. School nurses serve as health information resources and instructors both inside and outside the classroom.	❑	❑	❑
6. School health services provide counseling to address specific health needs as well as to reinforce positive health concepts.	❑	❑	❑
7. The health services/staff development programs provided to staff involved with health service effectively serve their continuing education/training needs.	❑	❑	❑
8. Parents, community members, and business representatives are satisfied with the quality and adequacy of the school's/district's health services.	❑	❑	❑
	(1 pt. each ✔)	(2 pts. each ✔)	(3 pts. each ✔)

COMMENTS:

_______ + _______ + _______ =
Total Column 1 Total Column 2 Total Column 3

____
Total Score

Comprehensive School Health Survey

School Environment

To what extent do the following statements characterize your school/district?

	Not Descriptive	Somewhat Descriptive	Very Descriptive
1. Decision makers within the district receive regular reports on school health issues and show strong support for CSH issues.	❑	❑	❑
2. People work as a team in assessing needs and in planning and implementing programs and activities in the area of comprehensive school health programming.	❑	❑	❑
3. The school/district has a tobacco-free policy on all school property for students and staff.	❑	❑	❑
4. The school is internally and externally safe, sanitary, and secure by the implementation of policies and procedures to prevent health problems and such things as tobacco, alcohol, and other substance use; violence; and vandalism.	❑	❑	❑
5. The school environment/staff development programs provided to staff involved with the healthy school environment effectively serve their continuing education/training needs.	❑	❑	❑
6. Vending machine items and other foods outside the cafeteria offer nutritious choices.	❑	❑	❑
7. The school staff (and central office) are open to suggestions and comments that could improve the school environment.	❑	❑	❑
8. Parents, community members, and business representatives are satisfied with the the school environment districtwide.	❑	❑	❑
	(1 pt. each ✔)	(2 pts. each ✔)	(3 pts. each ✔)

COMMENTS:

_______ + _______ + _______ =
Total Column 1 Total Column 2 Total Column 3

____
Total Score

Comprehensive School Health Survey

SCHOOL COUNSELING AND GUIDANCE

To what extent do the following statements characterize your school/district?

	Not Descriptive	Somewhat Descriptive	Very Descriptive
1. The school/district has clearly written and defined goals relating to school counseling and guidance.	❑	❑	❑
2. An adequate amount of staff time and personnel is allotted to the delivery and management of counseling and guidance services.	❑	❑	❑
3. Referral, coordination, and collaboration exists with other staff members and professional agencies in the delivery of counseling and guidance services.	❑	❑	❑
4. School counselors serve as health information resources and instructors both inside and outside the classroom.	❑	❑	❑
5. School counseling services provide counseling to address specific health needs as well as to reinforce positive health concepts.	❑	❑	❑
6. The in-service/staff development programs provided to staff involved with counseling and guidance effectively serve their continuing education/training needs.	❑	❑	❑
7. The counseling and guidance staff works collaboratively with other state and volunteer organizations.	❑	❑	❑
8. Parents, community members, and business representatives are satisfied with the school's/district's counseling and guidance services.	❑	❑	❑
	(1 pt. each ✔)	(2 pts. each ✔)	(3 pts. each ✔)

COMMENTS:

_______ + _______ + _______ =
Total Column 1 Total Column 2 Total Column 3

____
Total Score

Comprehensive School Health Survey

SCHOOL PHYSICAL EDUCATION

To what extent do the following statements characterize your school/district?

	Not Descriptive	Somewhat Descriptive	Very Descriptive
1. The school/district has clearly written and defined goals relating to physical education.	❑	❑	❑
2. An adequate amount of staff time and personnel is allotted to the delivery and management of physical education.	❑	❑	❑
3. Physical education includes daily activity in a K-12 program with a minimum of 15 to 20 minutes of aerobic exercise three times weekly.	❑	❑	❑
4. The physical education program is effective in improving or maintaining individual physical fitness in the areas of cardiovascular endurance, flexibility, and muscular strength and endurance.	❑	❑	❑
5. The school physical education/staff development programs provided to staff involved with physical education effectively serve their continuing education/training needs.	❑	❑	❑
6. The physical education program encourages and supports balance between competitive sports, physical development, and leisure skills.	❑	❑	❑
7. The physical education program encourages and supports individualized/adaptive fitness programs.	❑	❑	❑
8. Parents, community members, and business representatives are satisfied with the school's/district's physical education program.	❑	❑	❑
	(1 pt. each ✔)	(2 pts. each ✔)	(3 pts. each ✔)

COMMENTS:

_______ + _______ + _______ =
Total Column 1 Total Column 2 Total Column 3

____
Total Score

Comprehensive School Health Survey

School Food Service

To what extent do the following statements characterize your school/district?

	Not Descriptive	Somewhat Descriptive	Very Descriptive
1. The school/district has clearly written and defined goals relating to food service.	❑	❑	❑
2. An adequate amount of staff time and personnel is allotted to the delivery and management of food service.	❑	❑	❑
3. The cafeteria provides a clean and pleasant environment.	❑	❑	❑
4. The food service department plays an active role in the delivery of nutrition education, including point-of-sale nutrition information.	❑	❑	❑
5. The food service program coordinates health instruction with teachers to reinforce nutrition information learned in the classroom.	❑	❑	❑
6. The food service program models nutritional choices and behaviors, including the preparation and promotion of healthy dietary selections as outlined by USDA.	❑	❑	❑
7. The food service program provides appealing and culturally appropriate menu choices.	❑	❑	❑
8. Staff, parents, and students are satisfied with the quality and nutrition of the meals served.	❑	❑	❑
	(1 pt. each ✔)	(2 pts. each ✔)	(3 pts. each ✔)

COMMENTS:

_______ + _______ + _______ =
Total Column 1 Total Column 2 Total Column 3

____
Total Score

Comprehensive School Health Survey

Parent/Community Involvement

To what extent do the following statements characterize your school/district?

	Not Descriptive	Somewhat Descriptive	Very Descriptive
1. The school/district has clearly written and defined goals relating to the integration of school and community efforts to address health needs.	❑	❑	❑
2. The school/district offers activities to promote wellness among students, parents, and other community members.	❑	❑	❑
3. The school/district is open and encourages constructive comments from parents and the community.	❑	❑	❑
4. The staff, parents, and community members are satisfied with the means for disseminating and receiving information from the community.	❑	❑	❑
5. Parents, community members, health and human services representatives, and school staff members work together to encourage and support health programs and services for students.	❑	❑	❑
6. Periodic meetings are scheduled to collaboratively assess needs, and to plan, implement, and evaluate programs.	❑	❑	❑
7. The school and the community work collaboratively to solve problems by encouraging and supporting each other's health promotion efforts.	❑	❑	❑
8. Parents, community members, and business leaders are satisfied with the health programs and services offered by the school/district and those offered cooperatively with other state, county, or volunteer organizations.	❑	❑	❑
	(1 pt. each ✔)	(2 pts. each ✔)	(3 pts. each ✔)

COMMENTS:

_______ + _______ + _______ =
Total Column 1   Total Column 2   Total Column 3

____
Total Score

Comprehensive School Health Survey

EMPLOYEE HEALTH PROMOTION

To what extent do the following statements characterize your school district?

	Not Descriptive	Somewhat Descriptive	Very Descriptive
1. Administrators (school/district) support employee wellness programs, including the use of school facilities.	❑	❑	❑
2. Employees are satisfied that their needs and preferences are being met.	❑	❑	❑
3. Employees are satisfied with the organization and coordination of the employee health promotion program.	❑	❑	❑
4. Employee programs include health screenings and appraisals.	❑	❑	❑
5. Employee programs include educational/awareness programs.	❑	❑	❑
6. Appropriate follow-up of screenings, with referrals, and education is provided.	❑	❑	❑
7. The adult staff models good health and wellness behaviors.	❑	❑	❑
8. The employee health promotion program has an evaluation component including percent participation in programs and results of participation on records, absenteeism, insurance, weight loss, and so on.	❑	❑	❑
	(1 pt. each ✔)	(2 pts. each ✔)	(3 pts. each ✔)

COMMENTS:

_______ + _______ + _______ =
Total Column 1 Total Column 2 Total Column 3

____
Total Score

Comprehensive School Health Survey

STEP 2

INDIVIDUAL SUMMARY SHEET

COMPREHENSIVE SCHOOL HEALTH COMPONENT	SCORE TOTAL
• Health Instruction	
• Health Services	
• School Environment	
• Counseling and Guidance	
• Physical Education	
• Food Service	
• Parent/Community Involvement	
• Employee Health Promotion	

Give this summary sheet to the meeting leader so that totals for everyone can be calculated and the results can be discussed.

Comprehensive School Health Survey

STEP 3

Group Summary Sheet

Collect individual summary sheets from all team members. Then proceed as follows: (1) Assign a number to each summary sheet (team members are not to be identified by name); then enter the totals from all sheets in the spaces provided. (2) Total the scores for each component and enter the totals in the SUM column. (3) Divide the number in the SUM column by the number of individuals completing the survey, and enter the result in the AVERAGE SCORE column. (4) Divide the number in the AVERAGE SCORE column by 8 (the number of questions for each category) to get the AVERAGE RATING for each component.

Individual Scores

Comprehensive School Health Component	1	2	3	4	5	6	7	8	9	10	SUM (Total of All Scores)	AVERAGE SCORE (Sum ÷ by # of Respondents)	AVERAGE RATING (Avg. Score ÷ 8)
1. Health Instruction													
2. Health Services													
3. School Environment													
4. Counseling and Guidance													
5. Physical Education													
6. Food Service													
7. Parent/Community Involvement													
8. Employee Health Promotion													

Comprehensive School Health Profile

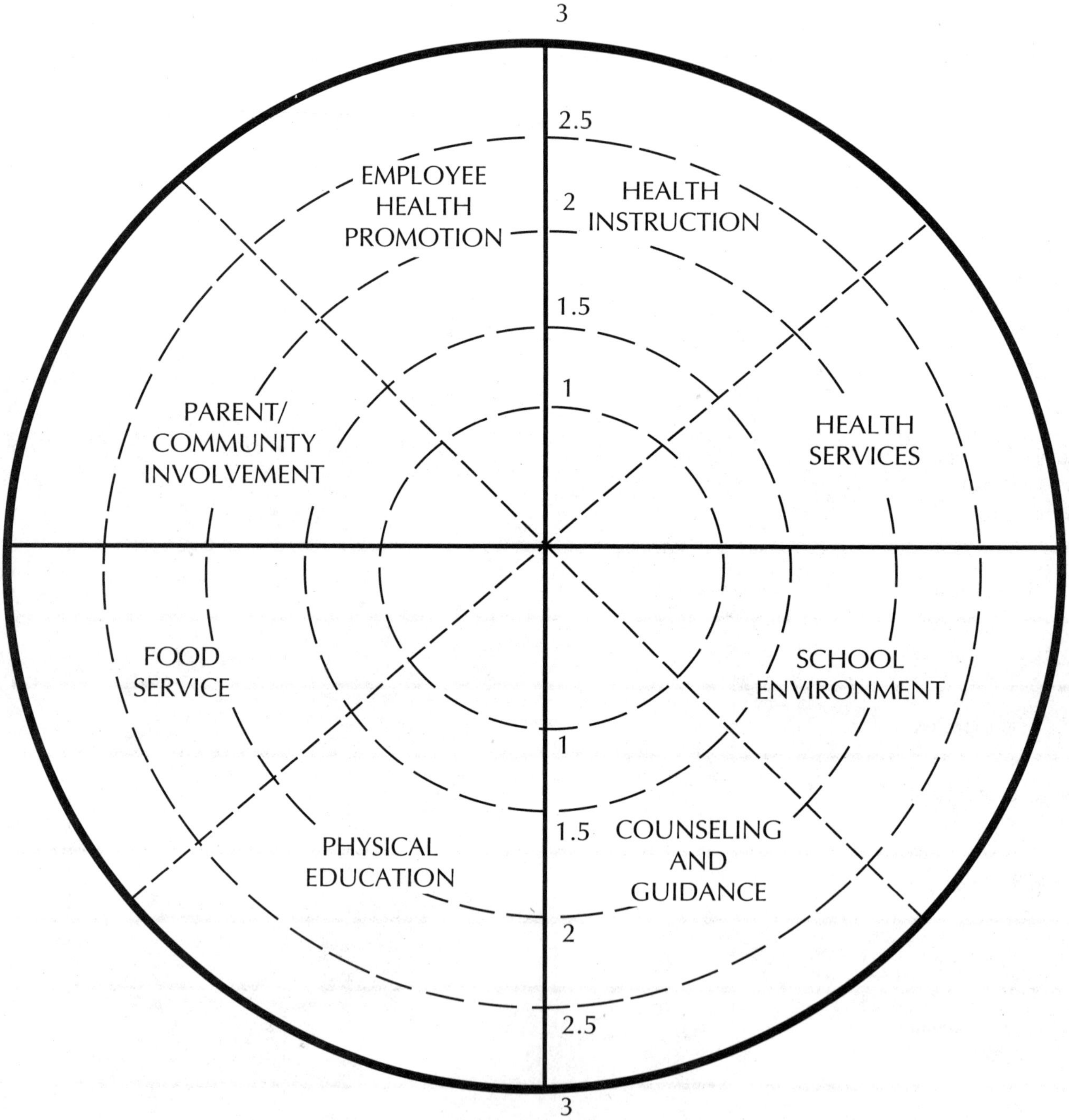

How healthy are your school health programs and services?

Appendix B

Sample Action Plan

Goal:

Objectives:

Action	Person(s) Responsible	Start Date	Completion Date	Evaluation Plan

Appendix C

Standards for Comprehensive School Health Programs

In general, school health programs and services are not guided by a unified, focused plan. Research has concluded that the multiple components of a comprehensive school health (CSH) program are traditionally delivered in independent and fragmented ways. In response to the need for clearly defined professional practices and desired student results relating to school health, one state (Texas) developed voluntary standards to help guide schools in their CSH efforts. A Delphi Review Process was used to define and make operable the following standards in an effort to assist schools in delivering CSH programs in a rational, collaborative, directed manner. The CSH standards may serve as the basis for developing needs assessment tools, outlining staff development plans, improving health instruction and services, and planning and evaluating programs. The voluntary guidelines developed through the Delphi Process are intended to be descriptive rather prescriptive.

The following standards are intended to serve as a model, or framework, for other states. Since their initial development, the CSH standards have been adapted by the American School Health Association for use as a set of national voluntary guidelines for comprehensive school health programming.

HEALTH INSTRUCTION

Policy and Administrative Support

- District policies and administrative guidelines reflect a commitment to attain desired student results essential to good health.
- The chief administrator and the school board receive, at least annually, reports on actions taken and results achieved.
- The board reviews, at least annually, its expectations for student mastery of desired student results.

Goals and Objectives

- District/school goals and objectives for health instruction are clear, based on assessed needs, and stated in terms of student results expected at each grade level and for each course.

Student Results

- Entry- and exit-level performance is defined for each grade level or health-instruction course.
- Formative and summative evaluations are conducted to measure appropriately student knowledge, attitudes, and behaviors related to health.
- Congruence exists between the evaluation measures used, the district's health instruction curriculum, and the critical health objectives for student learning.
- Students demonstrate mastery of essential health instruction objectives established for each grade level or course.

Curriculum

- Health curriculum content is targeted at priority areas appropriate for developmental stage and potential risk.

- Health instruction includes integration of the physical, spiritual, intellectual, social, and emotional dimensions of health as a basis of study in the ten content areas as suggested by the 1990 Joint Committee on Health Education Terminology: community health, consumer health, environmental health, family life, growth and development, nutritional health, personal health, prevention and control of disease, safety and injury prevention, and substance use and abuse .
- Health-instruction programs provide activities to develop decision-making and problem-solving competencies related to health promotion and disease prevention.
- Health instruction occurs as a regularly scheduled component of the curriculum at each grade level, and health issues are integrated regularly into almost every subject area.
- Teachers are familiar with the continuum of skills related to health for their grade levels or courses.

Teaching Methods

- Effective teaching methods are used to achieve the desired student results related to health.

Teaching/Learning Materials

- Current, theory-based, effective instructional materials are available to teachers.
- Staff education and training is provided in the use of all materials.
- There is coordination and use of available health education resources from agencies and organizations and others deemed useful by the local education agency/community (including but not limited to County/City Health and State Department of Health, Commission on Alcohol and Drug Abuse, Department of Mental Health/Mental Retardation, Department of Human Resources, American Heart Association, American Lung Association, American Cancer Society).

Parent/Community Involvement

- A committee that incorporates community representatives and parents, along with school staff, including teachers and administrators, operates in assessing needs, setting goals, and evaluating results related to school health issues and programs.

Staff Development

- Teachers are involved in identifying staff development needs regarding the teaching of health and working with school leaders to implement staff development programs to ensure achievement of state-recommended standards.
- Staff development and in-service training in current health issues and teaching techniques are ongoing and effective.
- At the secondary level, certified teachers with specialization in health are used to teach health courses.

HEALTH SERVICES

Policy and Administrative Support

- Policies and administrative guidelines reflect commitment to and accountability for an effective health services program.
- A unified plan exists to coordinate health services with other school programs.
- The district monitors and evaluates, at least annually, the health service plan, activities, and functions.
- The status of health services, including progress toward achieving annual objectives, is reported, at least annually, to the chief administrator, the school board, and appropriate agencies.

Goals, Objectives, and Program Results

- Goals and objectives for health services are clear, based on assessed needs, and stated in terms of expected results for students, faculty, and staff.

Student Services

- The planning, management, and delivery of school health services are supervised by a registered professional nurse.
- Screenings and immunization record maintenance of students are conducted as required by law (vision, hearing, spinal, and so on).
- School nurses provide direct, one-on-one instruction as needed and classroom instruction as requested by teachers and administrators.
- Physical assessment of students is made, including suspected child abuse, with appropriate health counseling and referral following.
- According to district policy, and upon proper authorization and orders, medication and direct health care services are administered to students by trained personnel.

School Staff Services

- Ongoing staff development and in-service training for faculty and staff, including health services staff, are provided.
- Registered nurses and other health-services staff provide resources and consultation concerning student and staff health issues.

Coordination of Services

- School health services are coordinated with community, city, county, and state agencies and organizations.
- To meet the needs of students and their families, school health services make use of available resources through professional and volunteer health organizations as approved by the chief administrator or designee in conjunction with the school board.
- The health services program, including a unified plan to coordinate health services with other school programs, is monitored by the district and used to improve program effectiveness.

School Environment

Policy and Administrative Support

- District policies and administrative guidelines reflect a commitment to maintaining an open and positive social climate with a healthy physical environment that is conducive to high student achievement and the long-term health of staff and students.
- The district receives, at least annually, a report on the social climate of the school and the workplace, and a report on the physical environment (water quality, sanitation in general, air quality, hazards, and so on).

Goals and Objectives

- The goals and objectives of the school environment component of CSH are clear, based on assessed needs, and stated in terms of intended results.

Social Environment

- Administrative support exists for a healthy social environment, as evidenced by district and school policies and procedures.
- The school environment is friendly, positive, conducive to learning, and open to new ideas and quality improvement.
- Problems are addressed appropriately and discussed openly within the limits of privacy.

- People work as a team in planning and implementing programs and activities.
- Employees and students are regarded as valuable and important.
- The focus is on people's feelings and needs as well as tasks and duties.
- There is strong encouragement for the staff to solve problems effectively.
- There is strong encouragement for the staff to deal with conflict in an open and respectful manner.

Physical Environment

- The quality of air, water, and other environmental elements is monitored to ensure the safety and well-being of students and staff.
- The school/district has a tobacco-free policy for students, staff, and visitors on all school-owned property.
- The structure of the building facilitates access by handicapped students.
- District and school emergency disaster plans have been established, and emergency drills are held periodically.
- Staff and students are regularly trained in emergency and first-aid procedures.
- Buildings and equipment are clean and kept in good repair.
- Student and staff comfort is maintained via adherence to adequate heating, cooling, ventilation, lighting, and noise standards.

School Counseling and Guidance

Policy and Administrative Support

- District policies and administrative guidelines reflect a commitment to and accountability for the social and psychological health of students.
- The chief administrator and school board receives, at least annually, status reports on the extent to which students demonstrate social and psychological growth and the extent to which identified student needs are met.
- Expectations for the counseling and guidance program are reviewed and updated at least annually.
- A unified plan to coordinate services with other school programs is monitored by the district and used to improve program effectiveness.
- There are an adequate number of trained counseling and guidance personnel, as measured by program effectiveness, to meet the needs of students.
- The counseling and guidance staff is effective in achieving the program objectives.

Goals, Objectives, and Results

- The goals of the counseling and guidance program are clear, based on assessed needs, and stated in terms of student results.

Direct Services to Students

- Counseling and guidance activities are effective in reducing inappropriate and unhealthy student behavior, promoting optimal mental and emotional health, and identifying and addressing problems.
- Guidance programming with students promotes problem solving, decision making, self-esteem building, and academic guidance.

Parent and Community Involvement

- Parents and community members, as evidenced by parental and community input, are satisfied with the counseling and guidance program.
- Programs are provided to assist parents and community members in building communication and other skills and in understanding child growth and development.
- The counseling and guidance staff uses available resources from the state, county, city, and volunteer health agencies to facilitate meeting student and staff health needs.

Staff Development and In-service Training

- The staff is satisfied, as demonstrated by effective support and programming, that the in-service education provided by and to the counseling and guidance staff addresses the multitude of mental health issues of children and adolescents.
- In-service programs are provided to assist with the implementation of guidance experiences that promote interpersonal development in students.
- All programs, including peer instructional programs, are organized to address health issues, including substance abuse, reproductive health, and mental health.

School Physical Education

Policy and Administrative Support

- District policies and administrative guidelines reflect a commitment to students' physical development and recreational skills, and to the promotion of lifetime health and fitness practices.
- The chief administrator receives, at least annually, a report on the status of students' physical fitness (strength, cardiovascular endurance, and flexibility).

Goals and Objectives

- School/district goals and objectives for physical education are clear, based on assessed needs, and stated in terms of student results expected at each grade level.

Student Results

- Entry- and exit-level performance for physical development are defined for each grade level and physical-education course, with adaptations made for students with physical, intellectual, or emotional disabilities.
- Evaluations are conducted to measure appropriately students' knowledge of physical development and recreational skills, and frequency and duration of participation in moderate to vigorous physical activity.
- Students demonstrate appropriate level of health-related fitness (for age and development as defined by AAHPERD, American College of Sports Medicine, and so on) and skills related to or needed for recreational activities for each grade level or course.

Curriculum

- Instruction includes integration of the physical, mental/emotional, and social dimensions of physical health.
- Students are involved daily in health-related fitness and recreation instruction at the elementary and secondary level.
- The physical education program is successful in encouraging and supporting lifetime fitness and leisure management.
- The physical education program has achieved a balance between sports and games and physical development.
- In addition to class time for skills instruction and additional activities, the physical education program provides opportunities for all students to have a minimum of 60 minutes of moderate to vigorous activity per week.

Teaching Methods

- Effective teaching methods are used to achieve the desired student results related to physical development and lifetime physical activity.

Staff Development

- Teachers are involved in identifying staff development needs regarding physical education and recreation.
- Staff development provided for the physical education staff is ongoing and effective in assisting students in achieving desired results related to physical fitness and recreation.

SCHOOL FOOD SERVICE

Policy and Administrative Support

- District policies and practices reflect a commitment to meeting the nutritional needs of students.
- Nutrition education is an integral part of the cafeteria experience.

Goals and Objectives

- The goals and objectives of the food service component of CSH are clear, based on assessed needs, and stated in terms of intended results.

Program Components

- Food service staff serve as a resource to teachers in providing nutrition education for staff (in-service) and students.
- The cafeteria is used as a nutritional learning laboratory.
- Students and staff, in general, are satisfied with the meals served, as evidenced by sales and meal consumption.
- Meals served meet USDA guidelines and recommendations for reducing the risk of chronic disease (i.e., lower salt, fat, and sugar content of meals).
- Meals served are sensitive to the ethnic and cultural food preferences of students.
- Candy sales for fund-raising are prohibited.
- Vending machines offer healthy food choices.
- Students are involved in menu planning.

PARENT/COMMUNITY INVOLVEMENT

Policy and Administrative Guidelines

- District policies and administrative guidelines reflect a commitment to effective parent/community involvment.

Goals and Objectives

- The goals and objectives of the parent/community components of CSH are clear, based on assessed needs, and stated in terms of intended results.

Program Components

- Continuing-education programs are offered for parents and community.
- Efforts are made to encourage parental and other community-member attendance (e.g., child care, evening meetings, coordination with other school activities, and so on).
- Two-way communication exists between school and community.
- A systematic means for sharing information, such as a community/school health advisory council, is in place.
- Periodic meetings, as determined by the local school or district, are held to assess needs, initiate recommendations, and evaluate programs.

- Integrated efforts are implemented to eliminate use of alcohol and other drugs, use of tobacco, motor vehicle injuries, sexually transmitted diseases, suicide, child abuse, teen pregnancies, eating disorders, and other health-related concerns.
- Evaluations are conducted at least annually to assess the level of satisfaction parent/community members have with CSH programs and services.

Employee Health Promotion

Policy and Administrative Support

- District policies and administrative guidelines reflect a philosophical and financial commitment to employees' health, including support for employee health promotion programs.
- At least annually, the employee health promotion program is evaluated and a status report is compiled and presented to the chief administrator indicating the kinds of employee health promotion programs supported by the district; the level of participation; provisions for quality assurance; and effects of health on economic factors, job satisfaction, absenteeism, and student behavior.
- An individual with appropriate training and skills is designated as the official manager of the employee health promotion program.
- The designated manager of the employee health promotion program receives administrative support via decision-making authority and is allowed time to manage the program.
- Employees are encouraged to model the healthy lifestyle expected of students.

Goals and Objectives

- The goals and objectives of the district's employee health promotion program are clear, based on assessed needs, and stated in terms of expected results.

Program Components

- The health promotion programs offered are based upon health assessment and employee preferences.
- Employee needs are determined by employees with input from health specialists.
- All employees are provided access to confidential health evaluations and screenings, basic education, and appropriate referrals concerning health.
- School facilities are made available for health promotion programs during noninstructional time.
- Employees are given adequate opportunities and incentives to participate in health promotion programs.

Appendix D

School Health Advisory Council Evaluation Checklist

	Yes	No
Does the school health advisory council (SHAC) or site-based decision making (SBDM) committee have a statement of purpose and goals related to student and employee health?	( )	( )
Do members have an understanding of what a comprehensive school health program is?	( )	( )
Has the council increased community awareness and support for school health issues?	( )	( )
Does membership reflect diversity of parents and organizations of varying and opposing viewpoints?	( )	( )
Does the membership include a broad-based representation of ethnic and economic groups in the community?	( )	( )
Does the group provide annual (at least) reports to the school board and other administrators?	( )	( )
Are members provided with facts and consulted when changes in the school health program are made?	( )	( )
Are resource materials on school health issues made available and used by members?	( )	( )
Does the administration seek and follow the recommendations of the group concerning school health issues?	( )	( )
Are meetings conducted in an open, impartial manner, allowing all members to express opinions?	( )	( )
Are decisions and recommendations of the group based on consensus?	( )	( )
Are meetings held on a regular basis at times convenient to a majority of members?	( )	( )
Do activities of the group support the mission and goals of the council?	( )	( )
Are objectives measurable, and are activities limited to those that can be completed in a realistic time frame?	( )	( )
Do the activities of the group support the ultimate goal of healthy students/healthy schools?	( )	( )

Adapted from Keith Howell, Dan Bibeau, Kathleen Mullen, Pat Carr, and Kathleen McCann, *Establishing and Maintaining School Health Advisory Councils: A How-To Manual For Local Education Agencies.* The University of North Carolina at Greensboro School Health Training Center, Greensboro, North Carolina, in cooperation with North Carolina Department of Public Instruction, Division of Curriculum and Instruction, Healthful Living Section, Raleigh, North Carolina, 1991.

Appendix E

Resource Directory

Many excellent materials, model programs, and resources are available to assist health educators in implementing health promotion programs. Without knowing where to look for these resources, however, health educators often "reinvent the wheel," spending untold hours of work recreating resources that already are available.

This resource directory is intended to help health educators easily find and utilize the resources they need. In fact, it is intended to help them find resources they didn't even know existed.

CODES

1. Aging
2. Alcohol, Tobacco, and Other Drugs
3. Chronic Disease Prevention and Control
4. Consumer Health
5. Care for Specific Populations
6. Environmental Health
7. Family Issues
8. Funding
9. Infectious Diseases Prevention and Control
10. Maternal and Child Health
11. Mental Health
12. Nutrition
13. Physical Fitness
14. Professional Associations
15. Public Information, Policy, and Regulation
16. Safety and First Aid
17. Comprehensive School Health Programming
18. Vision, Hearing, and Oral Health
19. Health Care
20. Worksite Health Promotion

Resource Directory

Organization	Codes	Description
Administration on Aging 330 Independence Avenue, SW Room 4760 Washington, DC 20201 (202) 619-0724	1	Government agency that assists in building community systems and assessing needs of the elderly.
Agricultural Research Service (ARS) Information Staff 6303 Ivy Lane, 4th Floor Greenbelt, MD 20770 (301) 436-7725	12	Government office that conducts surveys regarding the American diet; maintains the Nutrient Data Bank on the content of foods; provides dietary guidelines; develops materials on improving food selection.
The Alan Guttmacher Institute 120 Wall Street, 21st Floor New York, NY 10005 (212) 248-1111	10	Organization that conducts research, policy analysis, and public education in reproductive health.
Alcohol, Drug Abuse and Mental Health Administration Office of Communications and External Affairs Parklawn Building, Room 13C05 5600 Fishers Lane Rockville, MD 20857 (301) 443-8956	2, 11	Government agency that provides education on alcohol, drug abuse, and mental health.
Alzheimer's Association 919 North Michigan Avenue Chicago, IL 60611 (800) 272-3900	1, 3, 5, 7, 19	Association that offers referrals to local chapters and support groups: provides publications.
American Association of Retired Persons (AARP) 601 E Street, NW Washington, DC 20049 (202) 434-AARP	1	National organization that advocates for rights of older adults; maintains a strong network of local chapters; provides numerous educational materials, publications, and program support.
American Health Foundation 800 Second Avenue, 5th Floor New York, NY 10017 (212) 953-1900	17	Not-for-profit research organization for disease prevention and health promotion; offers school health promotion program called "Know Your Body," designed to help students develop skills for making positive health choices.
American Psychiatric Association 1400 K Street, NW Washington, DC, 20005 (202) 682-6000	11, 14	Professional association that provides educational materials.

American Psychological Association 750 First Street, NE Washington, DC 20002-4242 (202) 336-5500	11, 14	Professional association for the advancement of psychology as a profession and as a means of promoting human welfare; provides information for professionals and the general public.
Association for Worksite Health Promotion 60 Revere Drive, Suite 500 Northbrook, IL 60062 (708) 480-9574	13, 14, 19, 20	Association that integrates, unifies, and services a variety of interdisciplinary professionals for the purpose of influencing decision makers in the areas of health promotion/disease prevention and health care cost management.
Asthma and Allergy Foundation of America 1125 15th Street, NW Suite 502 Washington, DC 20005 (800) 7-ASTHMA (202) 466-7643	3, 4, 5, 6, 8, 15	Voluntary organization that provides general information, publications and videos, and physician referrals to the public; sponsors support groups, research grants, and professional education.
Center for Rural Elderly University of Missouri-Kansas City 5245 Rockhill Road Kansas City, MO 64110 (816) 235-2180	1	Organization that collects, catalogues and maintains a comprehensive database of information on progams, organizations, and resources.
Centers for Disease Control and Prevention (CDC) Public Inquiries 1600 Clifton Road, NE Mail Stop A23 Atlanta, GA 30333 (404) 639-3534	15	Government agency that provides information on a vast number of health topics including violent/abusive behavior, environmental health, unintentional injuries, and occupational safety.
Children's Defense Fund 25 E Street, NW Washington, DC 20001 (202) 628-8787	10, 15, 21	Advocacy group concerned with programs for children and youth; gathers data and disseminates information on key issues affecting children, including the development and implementation of federal and state policies.
Clearinghouse On Family Violence Information P.O. Box 1182 Washington, DC 20013 (703) 821-2086	7, 21	Clearinghouse that provides information regarding preventing family violence and assisting victims.
COSSMHO (National Coalition of Hispanic Health and Human Services Organizations) 1501 16th Street, NW Washington, DC 20036-1401 (202) 387-5000	5	Private, nonprofit organization dedicated to improving the health of the nation's Hispanic population; conducts research; provides information, policy analysis, and technical assistance; publishes *The Reporter.*
Doctors Ought to Care (DOC) Baylor College of Medicine 5510 Greenbriar, Suite 235 Houston, TX 77005 (713) 798-7729	2	Nonprofit international organization that promotes healthy lifestyles; emphasis is on educating children through humor about unhealthy products, especially tobacco.

Environmental Protection Agency Public Information Center PM-211B 401 M Street, SW Washington, DC 20460 (202) 382-2080	6	Government office that provides information about current programs and activities in environmental health.
ERIC Clearinghouse on Teacher Education One Dupont Circle, NW Suite 610 Washington, DC 20036 (202) 293-2450	17	Program of the Department of Education that indexes journals and research literature in database and compact disk formats on selected health topics; designed for use by teachers.
Food and Drug Administration Office of Consumer Affairs 5600 Fishers Lane (HFE-88) Rockville, MD 20857 (301) 433-3170	4	Government agency that disseminates information regarding nutrition and food and drug safety.
Food and Nutrition Information Center National Agriculture Library Building 10301 Baltimore Boulevard Room 304 Beltsville, MD 20705 (301) 344-3719	12	Library maintained by the Department of Agriculture that provides information on nutrition, food services, and food technology.
Funding Center P.O. Box 263 Alma, MA 04345 (800) 852-0001	8	Organization that offers specialized fund-raising assistance to nonprofit organizations.
Grantsmanship Center 650 South Spring Street Suite 507 Los Angeles, CA 90014 (213) 689-9222	8	Center that instructs public and private agencies in grantsmanship, program management, and fund-raising; publishes *The Grantsmanship Center's Whole Nonprofit Catalog,* a guidebook of resources for nonprofit organizations.
Head Start Bureau, DHHS P.O. Box 1182 Washington, DC 20013 (202) 619-0257	10	Government program that provides information on Comprehensive Child Development Centers and other Head Start Programs.
Health Promotion Resource Center Stanford Center for Research in Disease Prevention 1000 Welch Road Palo Alto, CA 94304-1885 (415) 723-1000	15	Center that provides technical assistance and support, videos, and printed materials on health promotion to public and private community organizations and agencies.
Health Promotion Resource Center Morehouse School of Medicine (HPRC-MSM) 720 Westview Drive, SW Atlanta, GA 30310-1495 (404) 752-1622	15	Center that disseminates materials and information on health topics, with special emphasis on low-income urban and rural minority populations; offers technical assistance to low-income communities in establishing health promotion activities.

Health Risk Appraisal Activity Carter Center of Emery University One Copenhill Atlanta, GA 30307 (404) 872-2100	15	Program that provides Health Risk Appraisal information and assistance in using the Appraisal through state and regional contracts.
Healthy Mothers, Healthy Babies Coalition 409 12th Street, SW Washington, DC 20024-2188 (202) 863-2458	10	Informal association of organizations with an interest in child and maternal health; fosters efforts to educate pregnant women; provides general information to health professionals and the general public.
Healthy People 2000 Public Health Service, DHHS Coordinator of ODPHP 330 C Street, SW Washington, DC 20201 (202) 472-5307	15	Coalition that developed the national Health Objectives for the Year 2000; provides baseline data.
National AIDS Clearinghouse Centers for Disease Control and Prevention (CDC) P.O. Box 6003 Rockville, MD 20849-6003 (800) 458-5231	9	Organization that assists health professionals involved with AIDS programs; provides technical assistance to organizations involved in the fight against AIDS; distributes publications.
National Alliance of Breast Cancer Organizations 9 East 37th Street, 10th Floor New York, NY 10016 (212) 719-0154	3	Coalition that provides unity among 300 organizations and individuals in the fight against breast cancer; serves as a resource, disseminates materials and information on support groups.
National Arthritis and Musculoskeletal and Skin Diseases Information Clearinghouse Box AMS Bethesda, MD 20892 (301) 495-4484	1, 3, 4	Organization that distributes patient and professional education material about rheumatic, musculoskeletal, and skin diseases.
National Asthma Education Program NHLBI 4733 Bethesda Avenue Suite 530 Bethesda, MD 20814-4820 (301) 951-3260	3	Program of NHLBI that works with intermediaries (such as medical associations, voluntary health organizations, and community programs) to educate patients, health professionals, and the public about asthma and related disorders.
National Cancer Institute (NCI) Office of Cancer Communications Building 31, Room 10A24 9000 Rockville Pike Bethesda, MD 20892 (301) 496-5583	3	Government office that distributes information about cancer and cancer-related resources; inquiries are handled by trained specialists.
National Center for Health Education in Maternal and Child Health 38th and R Streets, NW Washington, DC 20057 (202) 625-8400	10	Organization that provides technical assistance and develops educational and reference materials in a variety of topics related to child and maternal health.

National Center for Health Statistics 6525 Belcrest Road Room 1064 Hyattsville, MD 20782 (301) 436-8500	15	Center that provides professionals with assistance on the development of health measures; maintains library and distributes annotated bibliographies; distributes *National Health Interview Survey.*
National Cholesterol Education Program Information Center 4733 Bethesda Avenue Suite 530 Bethesda, MD 20814 (301) 951-3260	3	NHLBI program that has developed recommendations, guidelines and educational materials related to cholesterol.
National Clearinghouse for Alcohol and Drug Information (NCADI) P.O. Box 2345 Rockville, MD 20847 (301) 468-2600 or (800) 729-6686	2	Organization that provides the latest information on alcohol, tobacco, and other drugs in media formats including printed material and videos; publishes the bimonthly "Prevention Pipeline", resource guides, and a quarterly catalog. Maintains the Regional Alcohol and Drug Awareness Resource (RADAR) network centers in the U.S. and territories.
National Clearinghouse on Child Abuse and Neglect P.O. Box 1182 Washington, DC 20013-1182 (703) 385-7565 or (800) FYI-3366	7, 21	Organization that distributes publications and a free publications catalog; maintains a database of documents, audiovisuals, and national organizations; services include searches of databases and annotated bibliographies on frequently requested topics.
National Clearinghouse for Primary Care Information 8201 Greensboro Drive Suite 600 McLean, VA 22102 (703) 821-8955	5, 19	Clearinghouse that provides information to support the delivery of health care to areas that have shortages of medical personnel and services; materials include information on governing boards, financial management, sexually transmitted diseases, lead poisoning, administrative management, and clinical care.
National Coalition Against Sexual Assault (NCASA) 912 North Second Street Harrisburg, PA 17102-3119 (717) 232-7460	7, 15, 17, 20, 21	Voluntary organization with over 450 rape crises centers; sponsors annual conference; publishes current, accurate, and comprehensive sexual-assault related information to victim service providers, public policy makers, media, NCASA members, and the general public through *NCASA News* and the *Journal;* supports and monitors legislation on sexual violence.
National Committee for Prevention of Child Abuse 332 South Michigan Avenue Suite 1600 Chicago, IL 60604-4357 (312) 663-3520	7	Organization that publishes monographs, booklets, and pamphlets; provides research, training and technical assistance, and prevention programs.
National Council on Patient Information and Education 666 11th Street , NW Suite 810 Washington, DC 20001 (202) 347-6711	19	Council that provides information on programs, services, and materials that promote the safe use of medicines.
National Diabetes Information Clearinghouse (NDIC) One Information Way Bethesda, MD 20892-3560 (301) 654-3327	3	Agency of NIH that distributes publications regarding patient and professional education related to diabetes and its complications.

National Digestive Diseases Information Clearinghouse (NDDIC) 2 Information Way Bethesda, MD 20892-3570 (301) 654-3810	3	Agency of NIH that serves as a resource on digestive health; develops, identifies, and distributes educational materials; maintains an automated database.
National Eye Health Education Program Box 20/20 Bethesda, MD 20892 (800) 869-2020	18	Program of NIH; implements eye health education programs for the public and health professionals, including national campaigns and health education materials.
National Fire Protection Association P.O. Box 9101 Quincy, MA 02269-9101 (617) 770-3000	16	Association that provides technical information on fire prevention, firefighting procedures, and the fire loss experience.
National Foundation for Infectious Diseases/Immunizations 4733 Bethesda Avenue Suite 750 Bethesda, MD 20814-5228 (301) 656-0003	9	Nonprofit organization that supports research into the causes of and cures for infectious diseases; sponsors public and professional educational programs; provides postdoctoral fellowships for research; sponsors national awareness campaigns, and provides educational materials.
National Health/Education Consortium c/o National Commission to Prevent Infant Mortality Switzer Building, Room 2014 330 C Street, SW Washington, DC 20201 (202) 472-1364	10	Organized by the National Commission to Prevent Infant Mortality and the Institute for Educational Leadership to help better integrate health and education programs for children; provides a series of papers that focus on various topics relating to health and education.
National Heart, Lung and Blood Institute (NHLBI) Building 32, Room 4A21 9000 Rockville Pike Bethesda, MD 20892 (301) 496-4236	3, 9	Organization that provides national leadership for national programs and research related to the cause, prevention, and treatment of cardiovascular, pulmonary, and blood diseases; disseminates numerous educational materials for the public and health professionals.
National Heart, Lung, and Blood Institute (NHLBI) Information Center P.O. Box 30105 Bethesda, MD 20824-0105 (301) 951-3260 3, 9		Center of NHLBI that serves as the source of information and materials on risk factors for cardiovascular disease; disseminates public and professional educational materials.
National High Blood Pressure Education Program Information Center 4733 Bethesda Avenue Suite 530 Bethesda, MD 20814 (301) 951-3260	3	Center that provides educational messages to the public concerning high blood pressure.
National Highway Traffic Safety Administration (NHTSA) 400 7th Street, SW Washington, DC 20590 (202) 366-9294	7, 10, 16, 19, 20	Administration of the U.S. Department of Transportation that publishes brochures, flyers, statistical reports, videotapes, and other information about safety belts, and car seats; pedestrian, bicycle, and motorcycle safety; and drunk and impaired driving.

National Indoor Air Quality Information Clearinghouse P.O. Box 37133 Washington, DC 20013 (800) 438-4318	6	Organization that collects information on indoor air quality, including the health effects of passive smoke, formaldehyde, and various chemicals.
National Information Center for Children and Youth with Disabilities P.O. Box 1492 Washington, DC 20013 (703) 893-6061 or (800) 695-0284	5	Center that provides information on disabilities, legal rights, and advocacy; provides referrals and technical assistance.
National Injury Information Clearinghouse U.S. Product Safety Commission 5401 Westbard Avenue Room 625 Washington, DC 20207 (301) 492-6424	4, 16	Clearinghouse that provides data relating to morbidity and mortality associated with consumer products.
National Institute on Deafness and Other Communications Disorders Information Clearinghouse One Communication Avenue Bethesda, MD 20892-3456 (800) 241-1044	4, 5, 14, 15, 18	Clearinghouse that distributes information on hearing, balance, smell, taste, voice, speech, and language.
National Institute on Diabetes and Digestive and Kidney Diseases 9000 Rockville Pike Building 31 , Room 9A04 Bethesda, MD 20892-2560 (301) 496-3583	3, 12, 19	Institute of NIH that disseminates information and supports research on diabetes, renal disease, prostate disease, and other chronic disabling diseases.
National Institutes of Health (NIH) Division of Public Information Building 31, Room 2B-10 9000 Rockville Pike Bethesda, MD 20892 (301) 496-1766	1, 2, 3, 4, 5, 6, 9, 10, 11, 12, 15, 18	Division of NIH that provides information on a wide variety of health topics.
National Institute of Mental Health 5600 Fishers Lane 7C-02 Rockville, MD 20857 (301) 443-4513 TDD (301) 443-8431 FAX (301) 443-0008 FAX Information (301) 433-5158 Panic Disorder (800) 64-PANIC Depression (800) 421-4211	11	Government agency that provides information to the public, clinicians, and the scientific community with a variety of printed materials on such subjects as children's mental disorders, schizophrenia, depression, bipolar disorder, seasonal affective disorder, anxiety and panic disorders, obsessive-compulsive disorder, eating disorders, learning disabilities, and Alzheimer's disease.
National Institute of Neurological Disorders and Stroke Building 31, Room 8A16 9000 Rockville Pike Bethesda, MD 20892 (301) 496-5924 (800) 352-9424	3	Organization that disseminates information on the causes, prevention, diagnosis, and treatment of neurological disorders and stroke.

National Institute for Occupational Safety and Health (NIOSH) Technical Information Branch 4676 Columbia Parkway Cincinnati , OH 45226 (800) 356-4674	20	Federal agency responsible for conducting research and making recommendations for the prevention of work-related illnesses and injuries; provides publications, computerized databases, health hazard evaluations, fatal accident investigations, respirator certification, coal miner X-rays, training and research grants.
National Kidney and Urologic Diseases Information Clearinghouse 3 Information Way Bethesda, MD 20892-3580 (301) 654-4415	3, 4	Organization that is part of the National Institute of Diabetes and Digestive and Kidney Diseases (NIDDK); provides publications about kidney and urologic diseases.
National Mental Health Association National Prevention Clearinghouse 1021 Prince Street Alexandria, VA 22314-2971 (703) 838-7511	11	Clearinghouse that provides customized searches for current information on prevention of mental/emotional disabilities; promotes mental health through model programs, referrals and materials.
National Network of Grantmakers 2335 18th Street, NW Washington, DC 20009 (202) 483-0030	8	Organization that serves as a link for nonprofit agencies for sharing information and ideas on grantmaking; serves as a support network for organizations working on similar concerns.
National Osteoporosis Foundation 1150 17th Street, NW Suite 500 Washington, DC 20036 (202) 223-2226 (800) 223-9994	1, 3	Nonprofit organization that provides direct support for research; sponsors a national annual campaign; provides resource materials on osteoporosis for health care professionals and the public.
National Resource Center on Child Sexual Abuse 107 Lincoln Street Huntsville, AL 35801 (205) 534-6868 or (800) 543-7006 FAX (205) 534-6883	7	Organization that offers referrals for treatment and listing of professionals; provides assistance to communities; publishes a bimonthly newsletter.
National Resource Center on Homeless and Mental Illness 262 Delaware Avenue Delmar, NY 12054 (800) 444-7415	5, 11	Center that provides information and technical assistance concerning the needs of homeless, mentally ill people.
National Rural Health Network 1800 Massachusetts Avenue, NW Washington, DC 20036 (202) 857-4833	5	Organization concerned with the health needs of rural Americans.
National Safe Kids Campaign 111 Michigan Avenue, NW Washington, DC 20010-2970 (202) 882-4993	16	Program that provides informational materials to help increase awareness of the problem of childhood injury; designs programs to be implemented in communities to create a safer environment for children.

National Safety Council 1121 Springlake Drive Itasca, IL 60143-3201 (708) 285-1121	16, 20	Organization that deals with accident prevention, safety, and health in all areas.
National Stroke Association 8480 E. Orchard Road, #1000 Englewood, CO 80111-5015 (303) 771-1700 / (800) STROKES TDD (303) 771-1887 FAX (303) 771-1886	3	Association that serves as an advocate for stroke prevention, rehabilitation, research, and survivor support; offers a wide selection of audiotapes and printed materials for continuing education, staff training, and for the public.
National Sudden Infant Death Syndrome Clearinghouse 8201 Greensboro Drive Suite 600 McLean, VA 22102 (703) 821-8955	10	Clearinghouse that provides information and materials on SIDS, apnea, and other related issues.
Office of Disease Prevention and Health Promotion (ODPHP) National Health Information Center P.O. Box 1133 Washington, DC 20013-1133 (800) 336-4797	15	Government-funded agency that provides free publications and assists in the identification of resources regarding preventive services, nutrition, school health risk communication, and worksite health promotion.
Office of Minority Health Resource Center P.O. Box 37337 Washington, DC 20013-7337 (800) 444-6472	5	Government agency that disseminates information including reports, fact sheets, and database searches; provides technical assistance and referrals.
Office of Population Affairs Family Planning Technical Information Humphrey Building, Room 736E 200 Independence Avenue SW Washington, DC 20201 (202) 245-6335	10	Government agency that disseminates information on family planning and related issues.
Policy Information Center Department of Health and Human Services 200 Independence Avenue, SW HHS Building, Room 438-F Washington, DC 20201 (202) 245-6445	15	Center that houses evaluations and audits of DHHS projects, and reports by the Institute of Medicine and the National Research Council's Committee on National Statistics; descriptions are stored on computer-readable PIC database.
President's Council on Physical Fitness and Sports 701 Pennsylvania Avenue, NW Suite 250 Washington, DC 20004 (202) 272-3430	13, 17	Organization that offers presidential fitness awards and pamphlets on exercise, school physical education, corporate fitness, and other fitness topics.
Society for Public Health Promotion (SOPHE) 2001 Addison Street Berkely, CA 94707 (510) 644-9422 or (510) 845-4113 Fax	14, 15	National professional organization that promotes, encourages, and contributes to the health of all people through health education; identifies priority health issues; advocates on national and state levels; provides continuing education; supports training of professionals; publishes *Health Education Quarterly*.

Sudden Infant Death Syndrome (SIDS) Alliance 10500 Little Patuxent Parkway Suite 420 Columbia, MD 21044 (800) 221-SIDS	10	Private, voluntary organization to help families of SIDS babies; has a wide variety of information offered to the public; provides referrals for support groups and hospitals.
U.S. DHHS Region VI Office Division of Preventive Health Services 1200 Main Tower Building Room 1800 Dallas, TX 75205 (214) 767-3916	15	Regional office of DHHS that provides information on programs in the region.
Washington Business Group on Health 777 North Capitol Street, NE Suite 800 Washington, DC 20002 (202) 408-9320	20	Organization that provides information regarding current worksite health promotion programs in American corporations, including bibliographies of low-cost and free materials; provides lists of vendors offering services.
Wellness Councils of America Community Health Plaza 7101 Newport Avenue Suite 311 Omaha, NE 68152-2175 (402) 572-3590 / FAX (402) 572-3594	20	Organization that provides the publication *Healthy People at the Worksite 2000: An Information Kit;* supports community-based Wellness Councils, especially in worksite health promotion activities.

Toll-Free Numbers

Aerobics and Fitness Foundation	1-800-233-4886
AIDS Clinical Trials Information Service	1-800-874-2572
AIDS Legal Assistance Line	1-800-828-6417
Alzheimer's Disease and Related Disorders (National)	1-800-621-0379
American Cancer Society	1-800-ACS-2345
American Diabetes Association	1-800-232-3472
American Lung Association	1-800-252-LUNG
Arthritis Foundation Information Line	1-800-283-7800
Asthma and Allergy Foundation	1-800-7ASTHMA
Battered Women National Hotline	1-800-333-7233
BABYLOVE Information Line (prenatal and infant care)	1-800-4BABYLOVE
Boystown Suicide Hotline	1-800-448-3000
Cancer Information Service (MD Anderson)	1-800-4CANCER
Cancer Research Nutrition Hotline	1-800-843-8114
Child Abuse Report to DHS (24-hour)	1-800-252-5400
Child Find/Missing Children	1-800-426-5678
Childhelp USA (counseling, referral)	1-800-4-A-CHILD
Cocaine Hotline (24-hour)	1-800-COCAINE
Covenant House National 9 Line (runaways, others)	1-800-999-9999
Drug and Alcohol Abuse/Eating Disorders/Gay Issues	1-800-444-9999
HUD Drug Information Clearinghouse	1-800-245-2691
Juvenile Diabetes Foundation Hotline	1-800-223-1138
Medicare Telephone Hotline	1-800-638-6833
National AIDS Hotline	1-800-342-AIDS
National AIDS Hotline—Spanish	1-800-344-SIDA
National AIDS Information Clearinghouse	1-800-458-5231
National Clearinghouse on Alcohol and Drug Information.	1-800-SAY-NOTO
National Clearinghouse on Child Abuse and Neglect	1-800-FYI-3366
National Clearinghouse on Family Support	1-800-628-1696
National Commission on Alcoholism and Drug Dependence	1-800-475-HOPE
National Council on Aging	1-800-424-9046
National Council on Alcoholism and Drug Dependence	1-800-NCA-CALL
National Eye Health Education Program, NIH	1-800-869-2020
National Health Information Center	1-800-336-4797
National Hospice Organization	1-800-658-8898
National Indoor Air Quality Information Center	1-800-438-4318
National Information Center for Children with Disabilities	1-800-999-5599
National Institute on Deafness Information Clearinghouse	1-800-241-1044
National Institute on Drug Abuse Hotline	1-800-662-HELP
National Marrow Donor Program	1-800-654-1247
National Migrant Resource Program	1-800-531-5120
National Pediatric HIV Resource Center	1-800-362-0071
National Resource Center—Homelessness and Mental Illness	1-800-444-7415
National Runaway Switchboard	1-800-621-4000
National Sexually Transmitted Diseases Hotline	1-800-227-8922
National Stroke Association	1-800-STROKES
National Youth Crisis Hotline	1-800-448-4663
ODPHP National Health Information Center	1-800-336-4797
Office of Minority Health Resource Center	1-800-444-MHRC
Office of Substance Abuse Prevention	1-800-729-6686
Runaway Hotline	1-800-392-3352

Safe Rider Program (child passenger safety)	1-800-252-8255
Senior Citizens' Occupant Protection Program	1-800-252-8255
Sudden Infant Death Syndrome (SIDS) Alliance	1-800-221-SIDS
Susan B. Komen Foundation (breast cancer information)	1-800-462-9273
TARGET (alcohol and drug prevention)	1-800-366-6667
Team Challenge (drug/alcohol)	1-800-727-0508
Teens TAP (Teaching AIDS Prevention)	1-800-234-TEEN
Women's Domestic Violence Center	1-800-441-5555
Y-ME Breast Cancer Support Program	1-800-221-2141

Bibliography

1. *Kids Count Data Book.* Greenwich, CN: Annie E. Casey Foundation, 1994, p. 14.
2. Texas Department of Corrections. Telephone interview, May 1992.
3. Texas Higher Education Coordinating Board. Telephone interview, May 1992.
4. Gans, JE, MA McManus, and PW Newacheck, (eds.). *Adolescent Health Care: Use, Costs, and Problems of Access,* Vol. 2 in AMA Profiles of Adolescent Health Series. Chicago, IL: American Medical Association, 1991, pp. x, 42.
5. Allensworth, DD, and LJ Kolbe. "The Comprehensive School Health Program: Exploring an Expanded Concept." *J Sch Health.* 57:10 (1987), 409–412.
6. *Healthy People 2000: National Health Promotion and Disease Prevention Objectives.* Washington, DC: Public Health Service, DHHS Office of the Assistant Secretary for Health, 1990.
7. *Chronic Disease and Health Promotion Reprints from the MMWR, 1990–1991 Youth Risk Behavior Surveillance System.* Atlanta, GA: U.S. Department of Health and Human Services, Centers for Disease Control and Prevention, 1992, pp. 15, 25.
8. *Code Blue: Uniting for Healthier Youth.* Alexandria, VA: National Association of State Boards of Education and American Medical Association, 1990, pp. 3, 4.
9. Center for Population Options. Telephone interview, December 1994.
10. Center for Population Options. *Adolescents, HIV and Other Sexually Transmitted Diseases.* Washington, DC: , May 1993.
11. Cortese, P, and K Middleton (eds.). *The Comprehensive School Health Challenge,* Vol. 1. Santa Cruz, CA: ETR Associates, 1994, p. 4.
12. Center for the Study of Social Policy. *The National Education Goals Report: Building a Nation of Learners.* Washington, DC: U.S. Government Printing Office, 1992, p. 76.

Credits

This book began as a project of the Texas Comprehensive School Health Initiative, a voluntary consortium of more than 25 health- and education-related organizations that is administered by the Texas Association of School Administrators. The mission of TCSHI is to "promote and enhance the health and well-being of Texas children, youth, and their families through a collaborative effort between Texas organizations and schools." The authors wish to acknowledge consortium members representing the following organizations and agencies who have supported the continuing development of the tools and materials contained in this document:

AIDS Consortium of Texas — Colleges and Universities
American Cancer Society
American Heart Association
American Lung Association
Association of Texas Professional Educators
Center for Public Policy Priorities
Fort Worth Independent School District
Governor's Commission on Physical Fitness
March of Dimes Birth Defects Foundation
National Health/Education Consortium
Texas Association for Health, Physical Education, Recreation, and Dance
Texas Association of School Administrators
Texas Association of School Boards
Texas Association of Secondary School Principals
Texas Cancer Council
Texas Commission on Alcohol and Drug Abuse
Texas Congress of Parents and Teachers
Texas Department of Health
Texas Department of Human Services
Texas Department of Mental Health/Mental Retardation
Texas Dietetic Association
Texas Education Agency
Texas Elementary Principals and Supervisors Association
Texas Family Planning Association
Texas Medical Association
Texas Mental Health Association
Texas Prevention Partnership
Texas School Counselors Association
Texas School Food Services Association
Texas School Health Association
Texas School Nurses Association
Texas School Public Relations Association
University of Texas at Austin
University of Texas Health Science Center at Houston

In addition to the work of the consortium members, the authors wish to extend thanks to members of the Delphi panel who assisted in the development of the CSH standards found in Appendix C. Delphi panel members included:

Diane Allensworth, American School Health Association
Judy Baker, Texas Woman's University
Danny Ballard, Texas A&M University
Joel Barton, Lamar University
Steve Furney, Southwest Texas State University
Don Haydon, University of Texas at Austin
Henry Herrera, Alice ISD
Nick Iammarino, Rice University
Mary Jackson, Texas Education Agency
Gay James, Southwest Texas State University
Stephen Maldonado, Northside ISD
Jane McDonald, American Association of School Administrators
Brenda Mitchell, Institute for Aerobics Research
Guy Parcel, University of Texas Health Science Center, Houston
Rusty Pippin, Baylor University
Buzz Pruitt, Texas A&M University
Roger Rodriguez, San Antonio ISD
Shirley Schreiber, Texas Association of School Nurses
Sunny Thomas Allcorn, TEA-Comprehensive School Health
Len Tritsch, American Association of School Administrators
Sherry Woodard, Silsbee ISD
Roberto Zamora, La Joya ISD

Appreciation is also given to Jill Fielder Brown, who co-authored the original resource directory, and Sarah Olson from the Texas Department of Health, Division of Public Health Promotion, for co-authoring and updating the resource directory found in Appendix E.

Finally, special appreciation is extended to the Texas Association of School Administrators, National Health/Education Consortium, AT&T Foundation, and the U.S. Department of Education, Office of Educational Research and Improvement, for funding the development of the Texas document, which has since been edited for this national distribution. Opinions expressed in this document and the Texas publication do not necessarily reflect the views of the supporting organizations and agencies, individual consortium members, or funders.

Notes

Notes

Notes

Notes